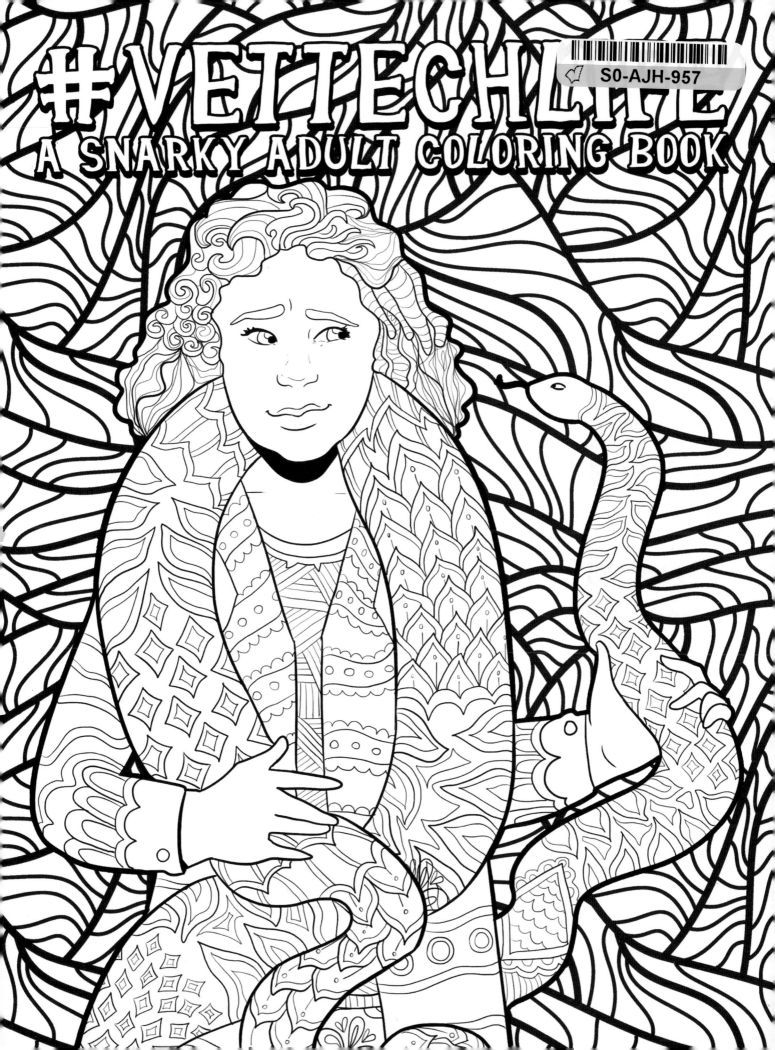

#VETTECHLIFE
A SNARKY ADULT COLORING BOOK

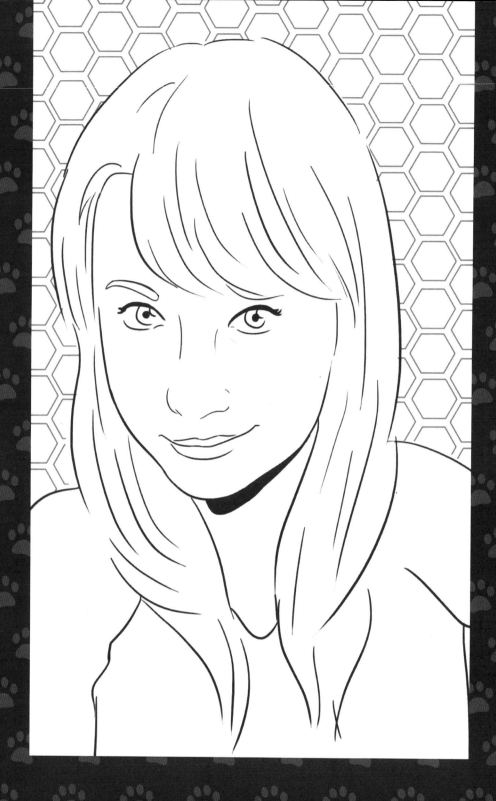

Illustrated by Micaela

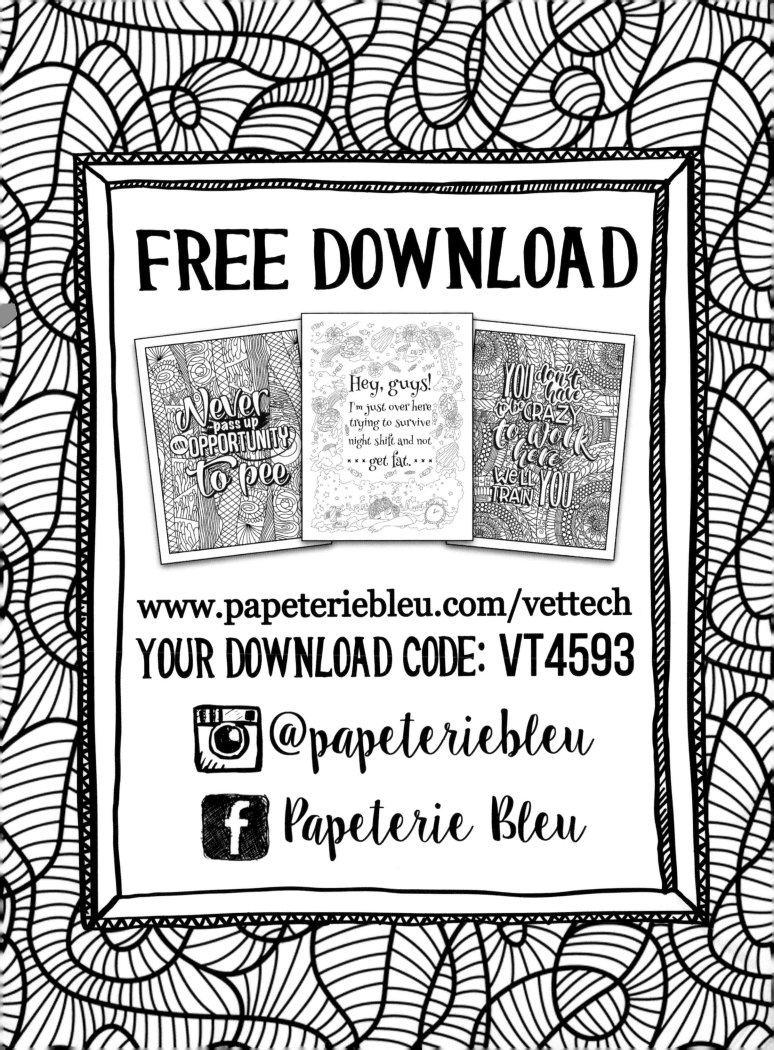

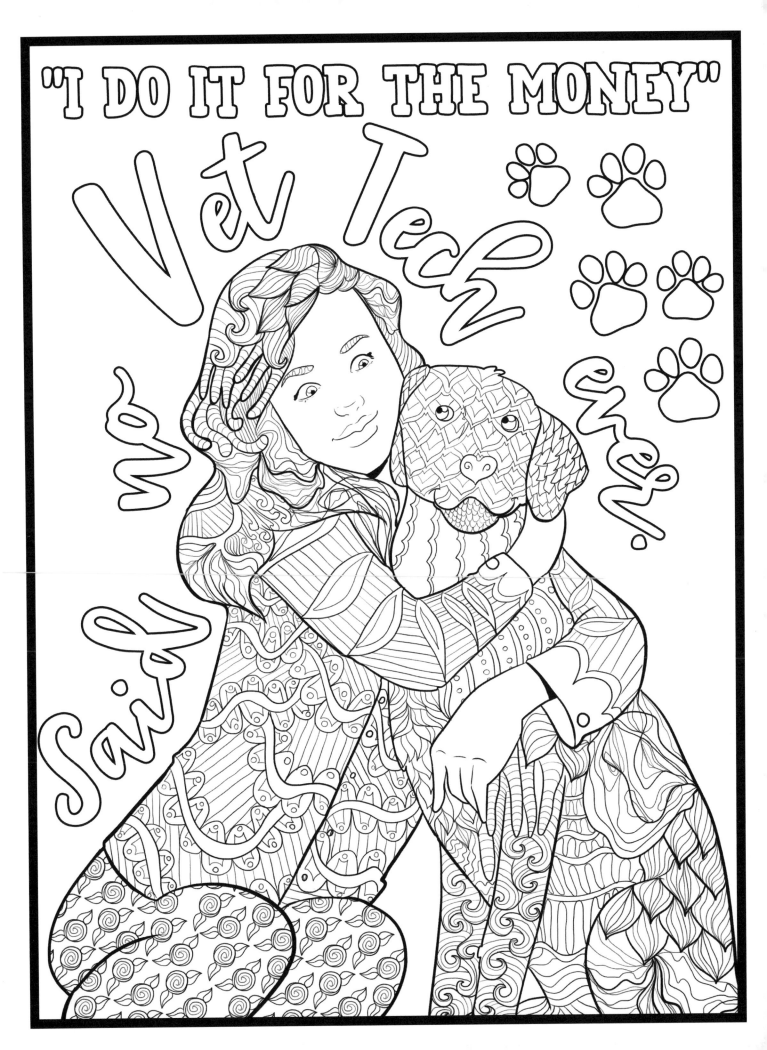

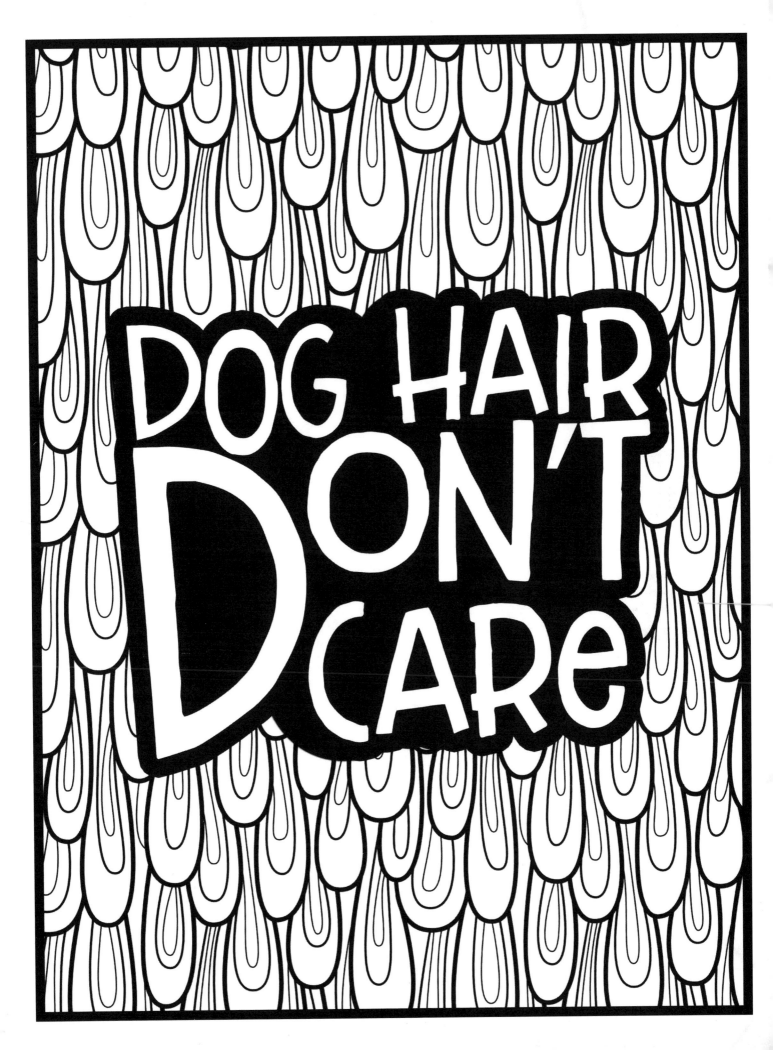

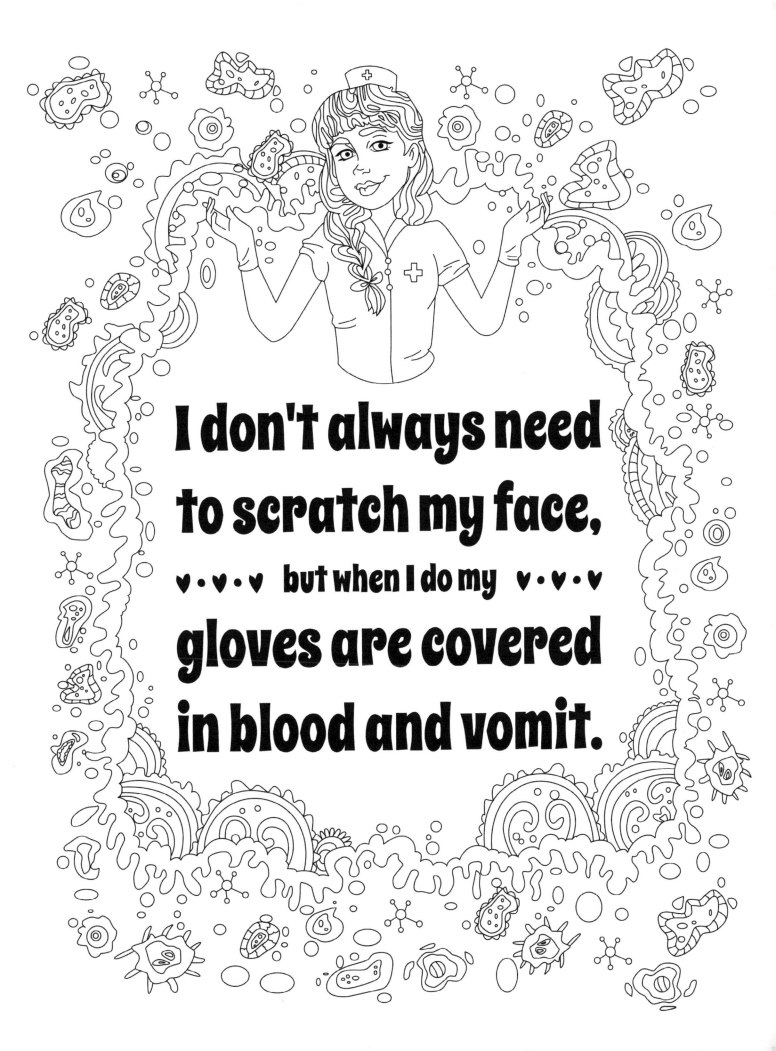

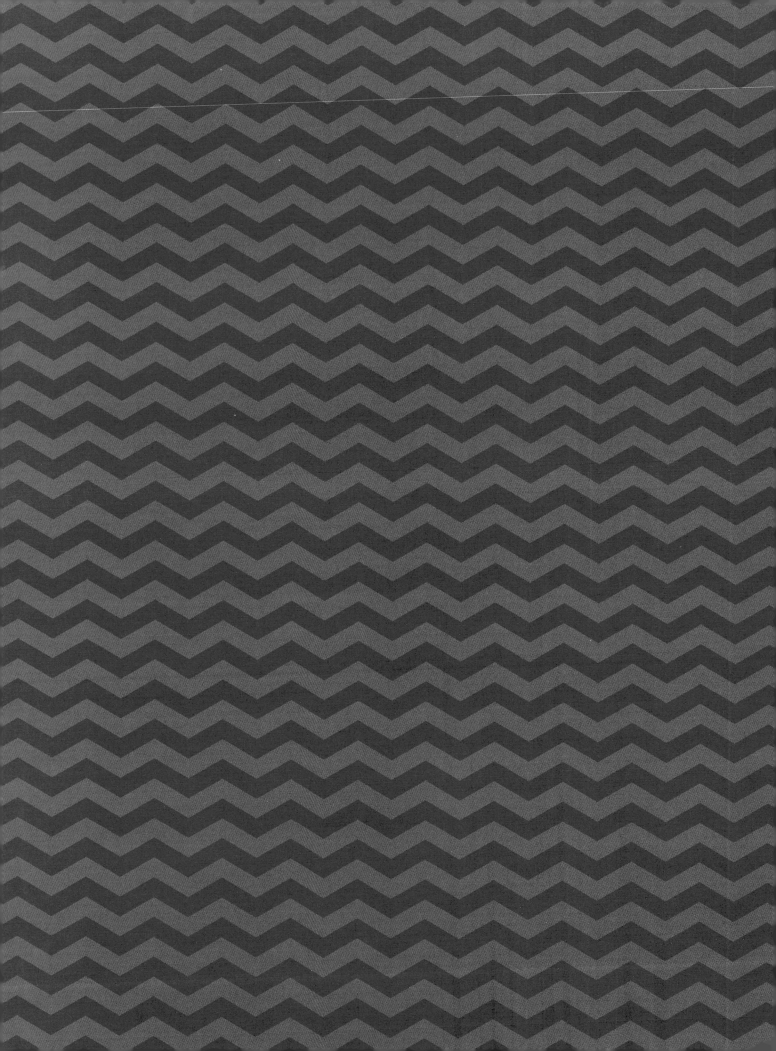

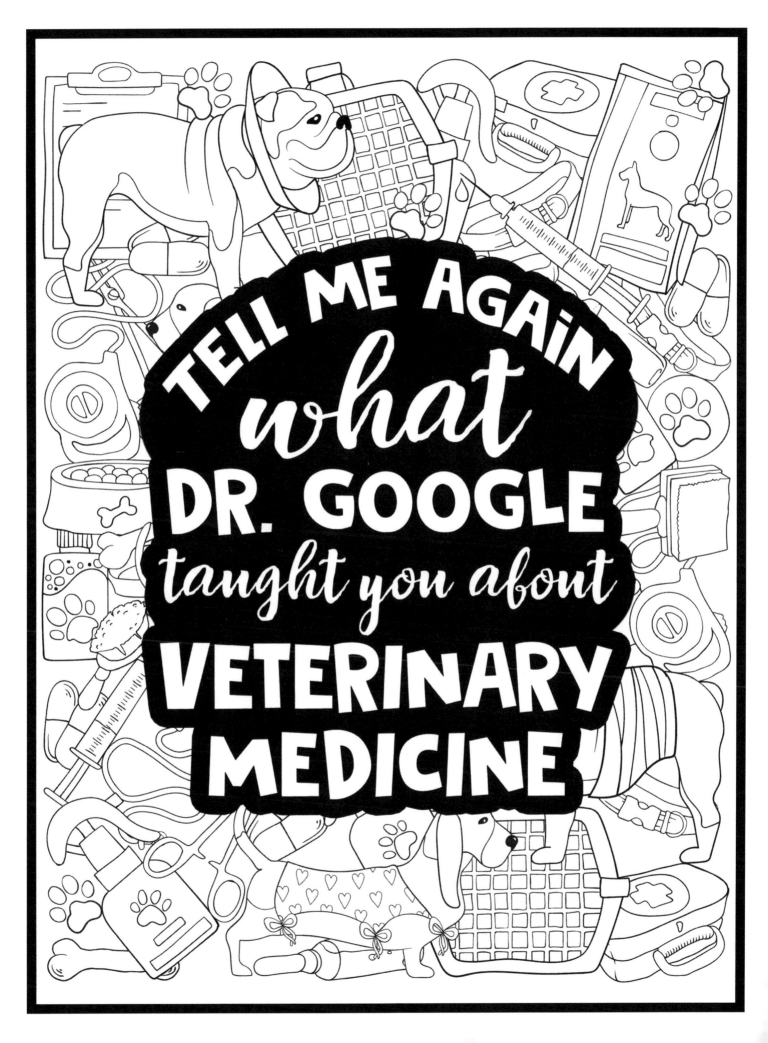

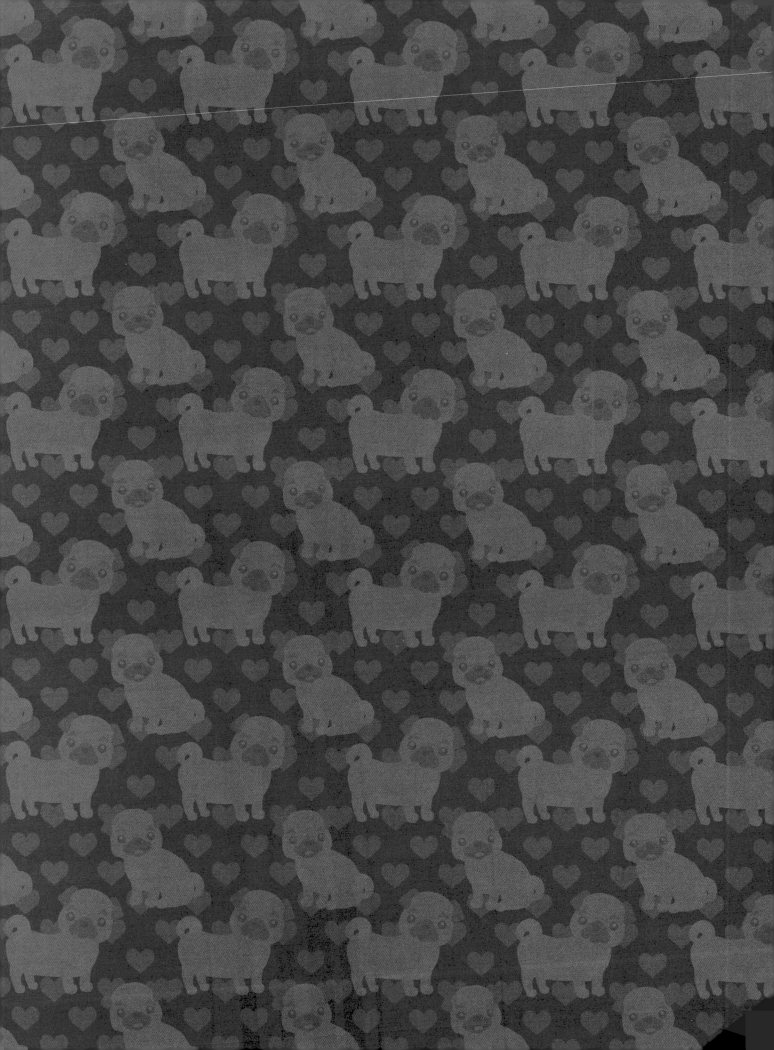

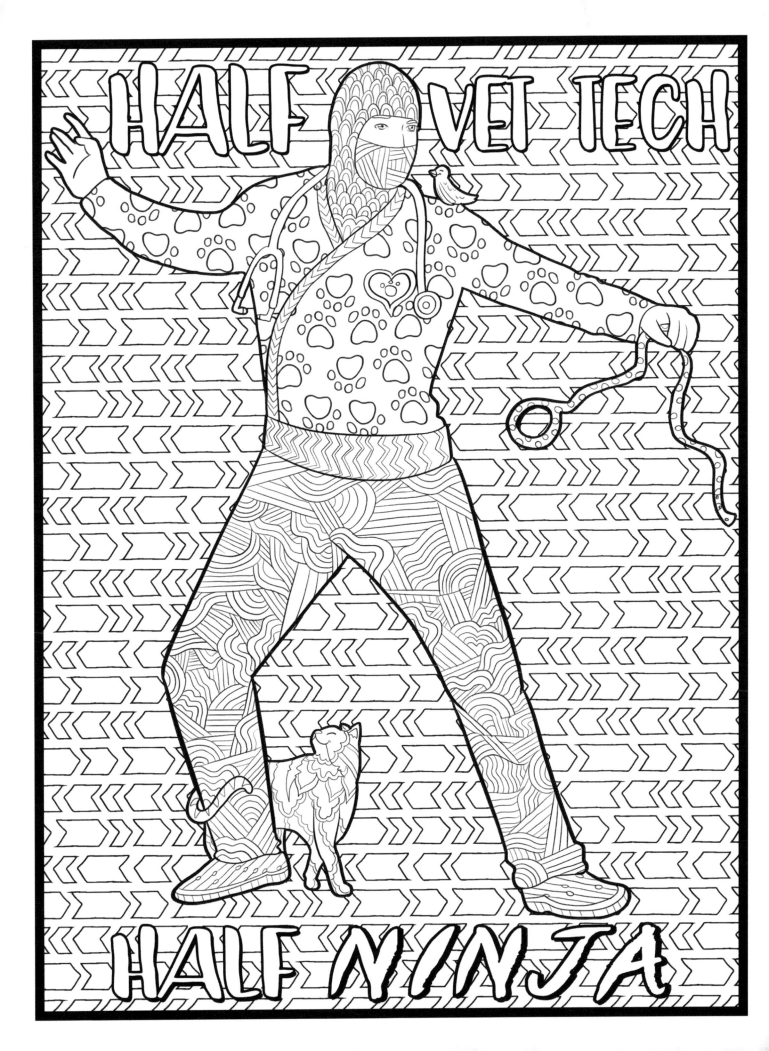

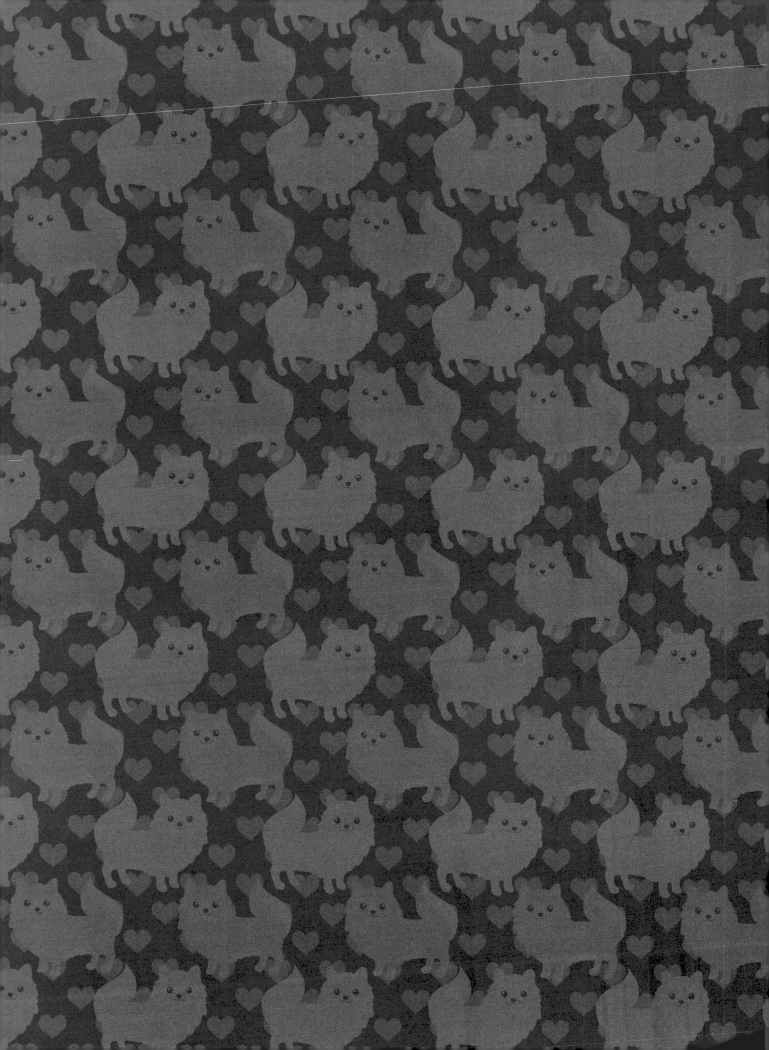

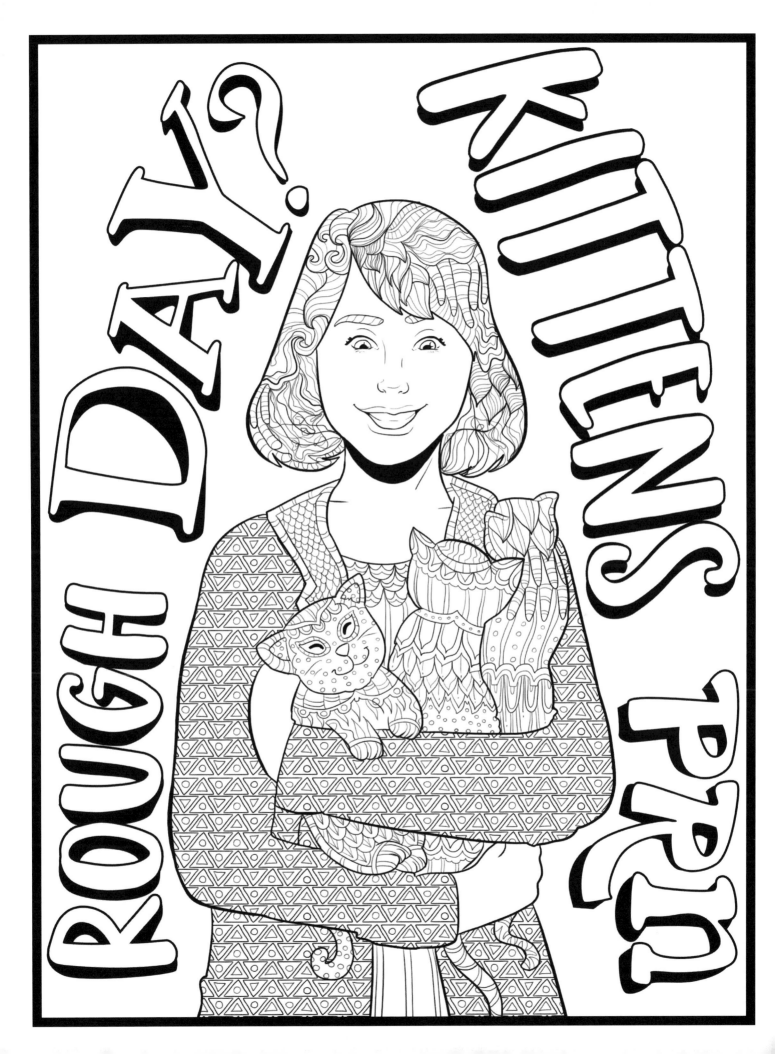

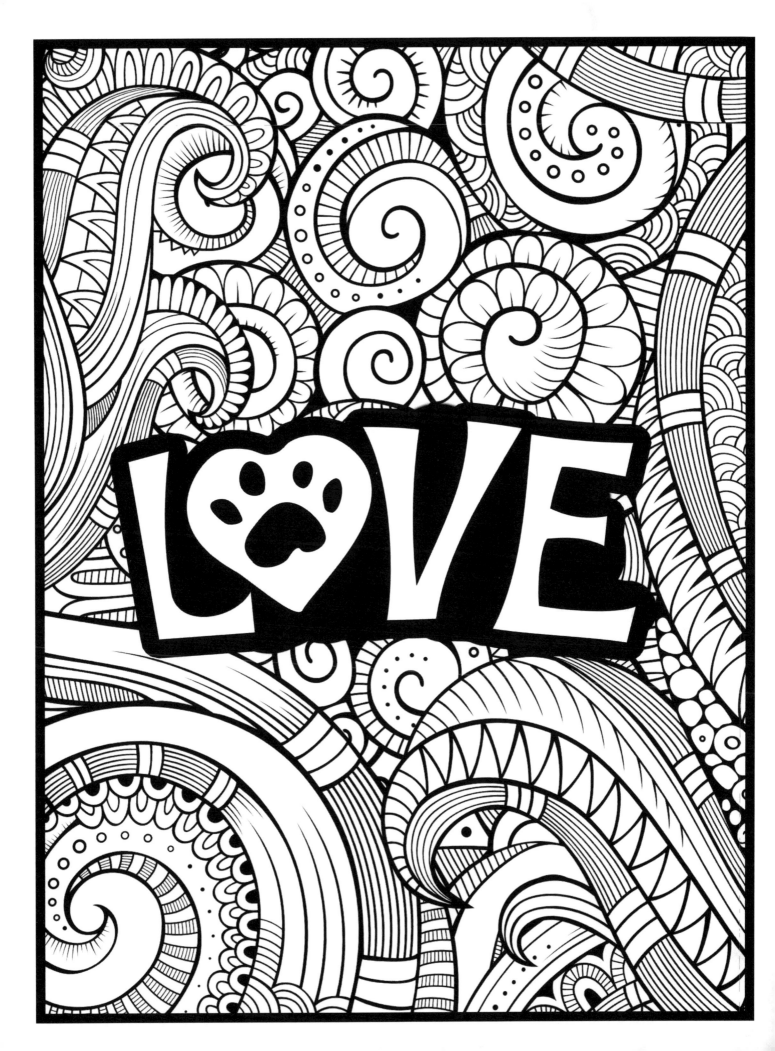

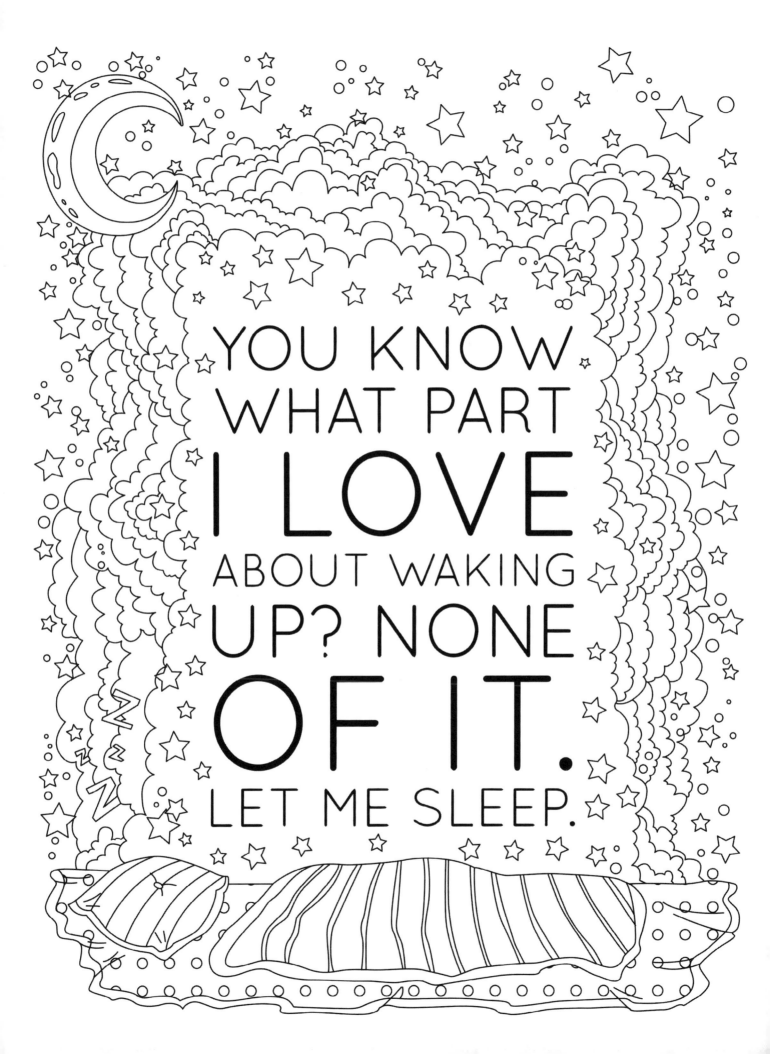

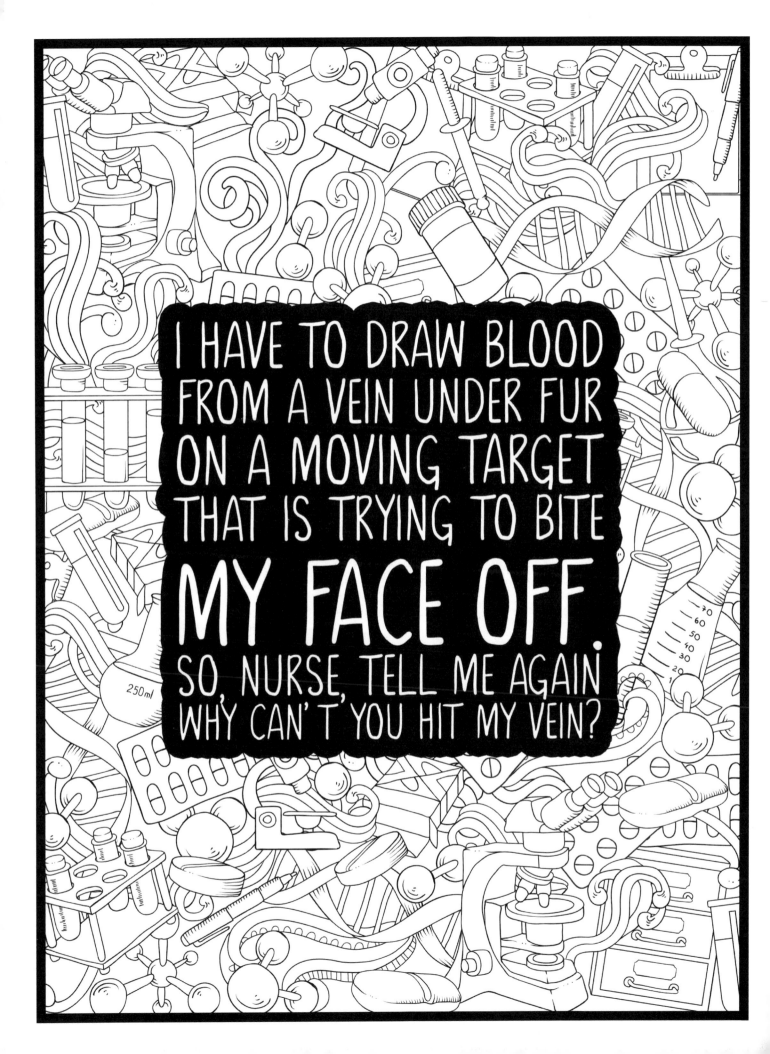

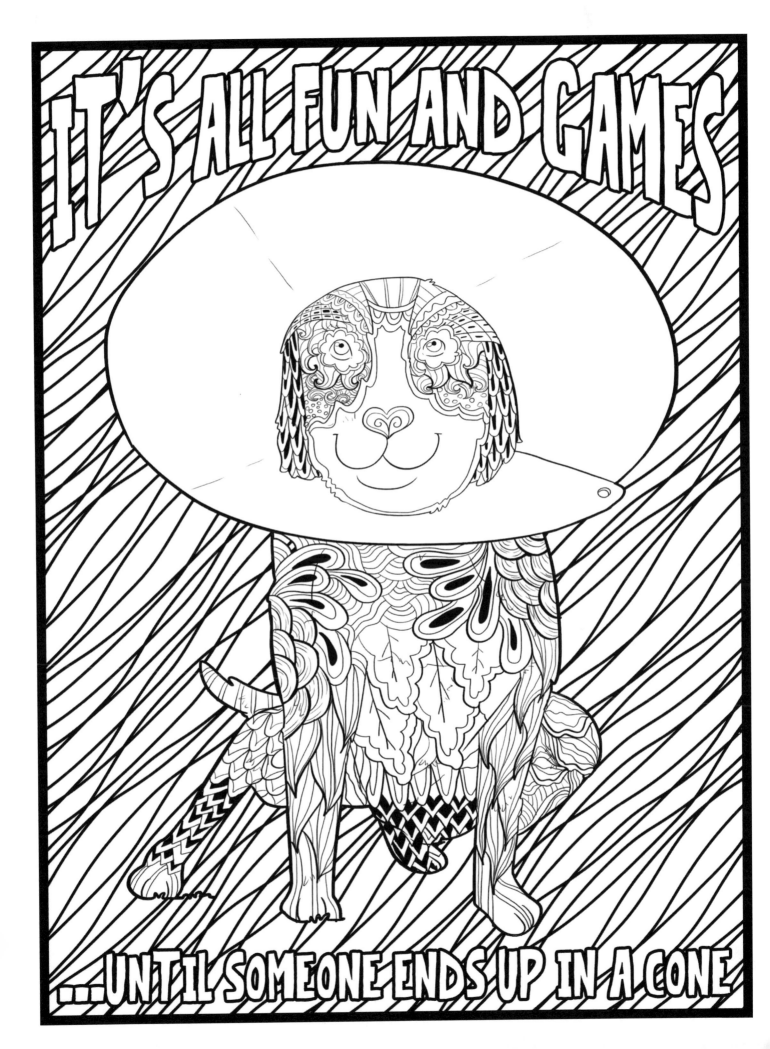

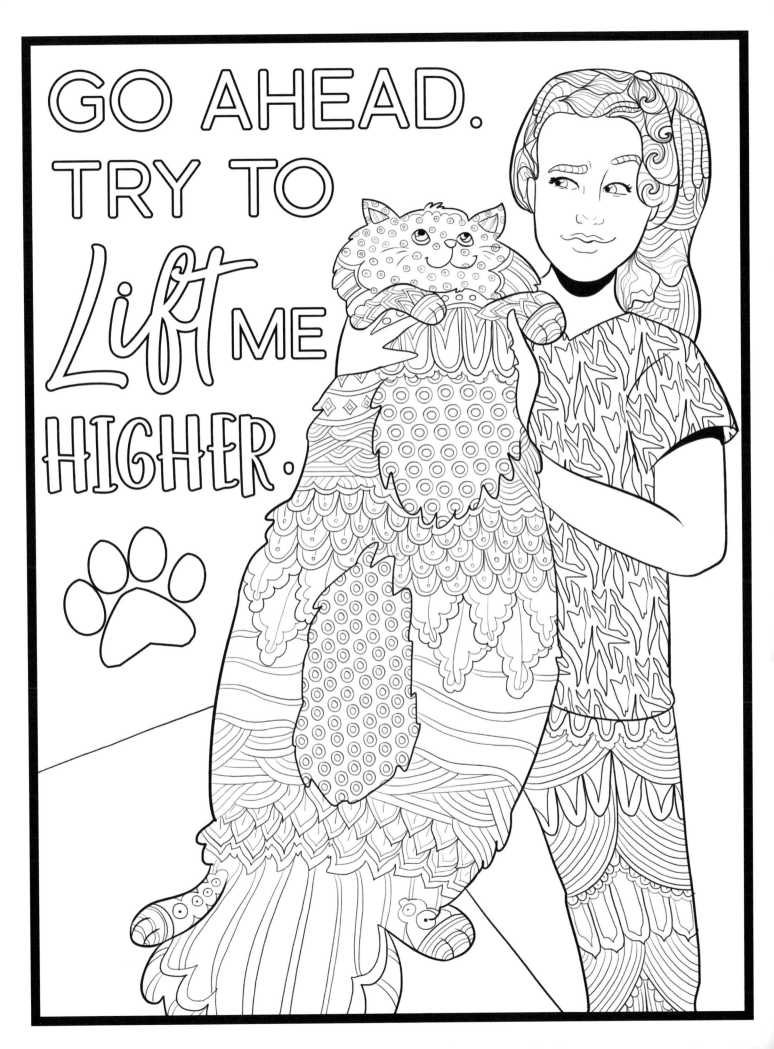

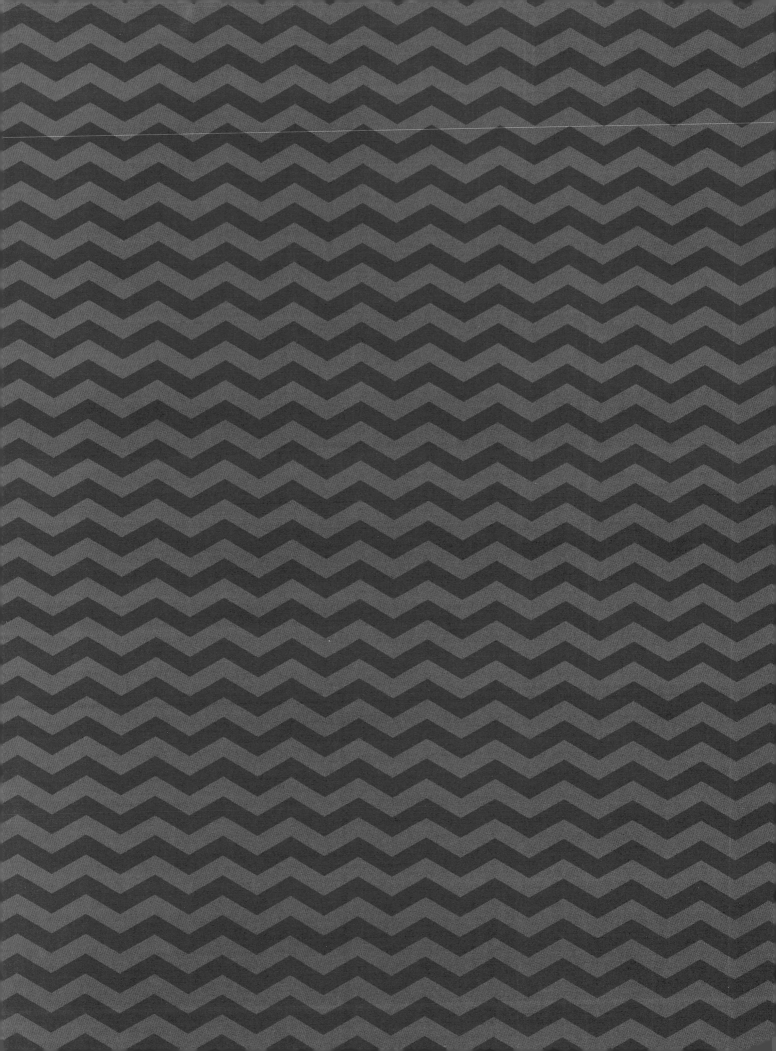

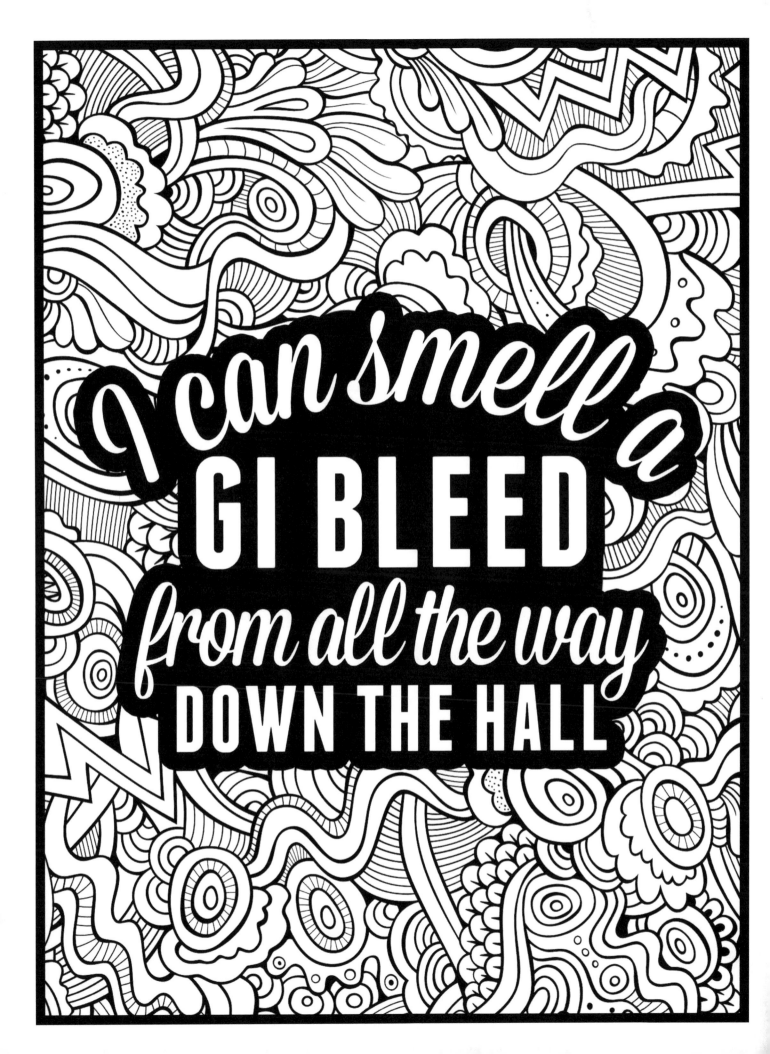

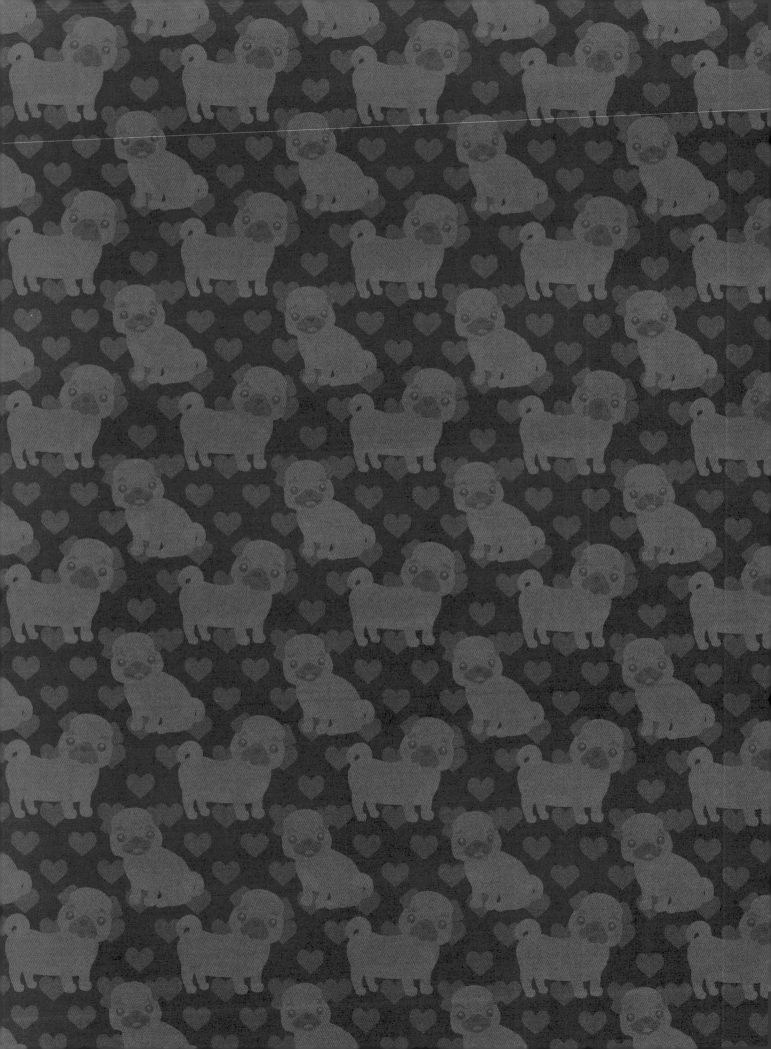

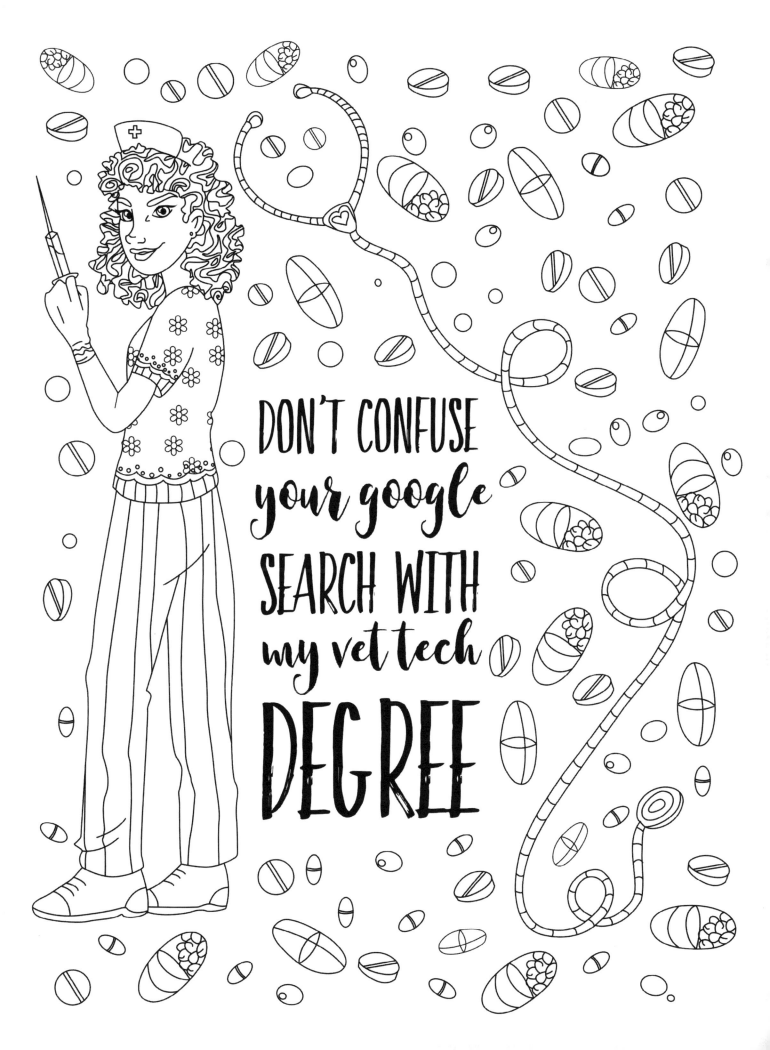

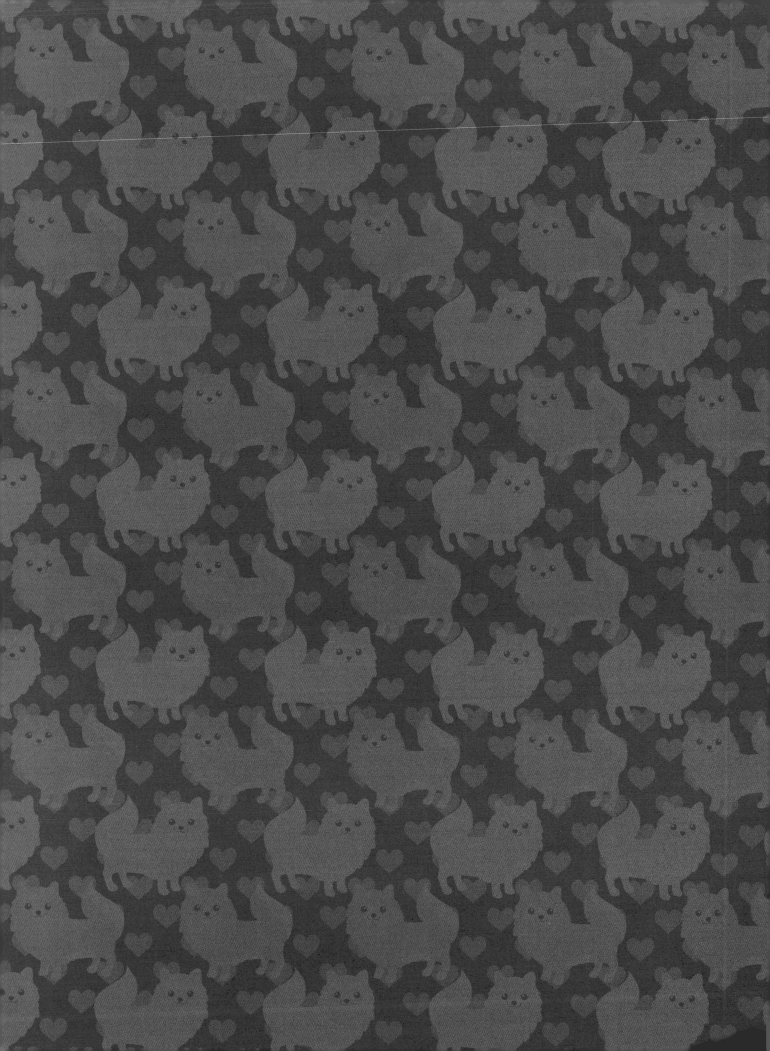

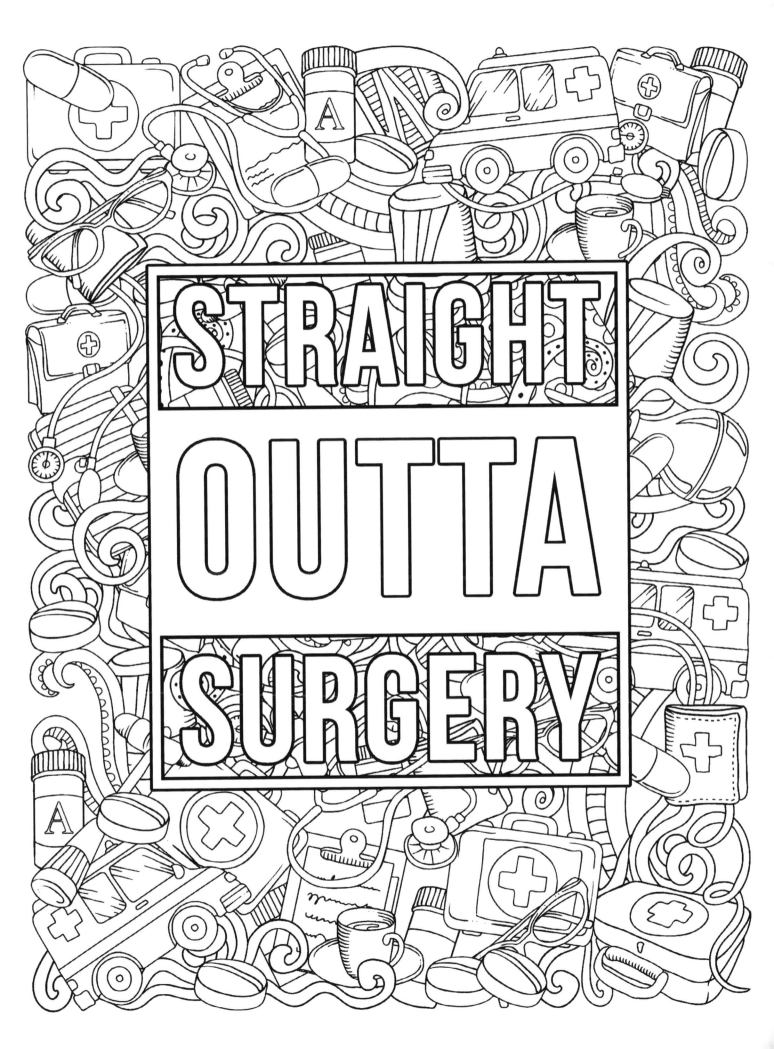

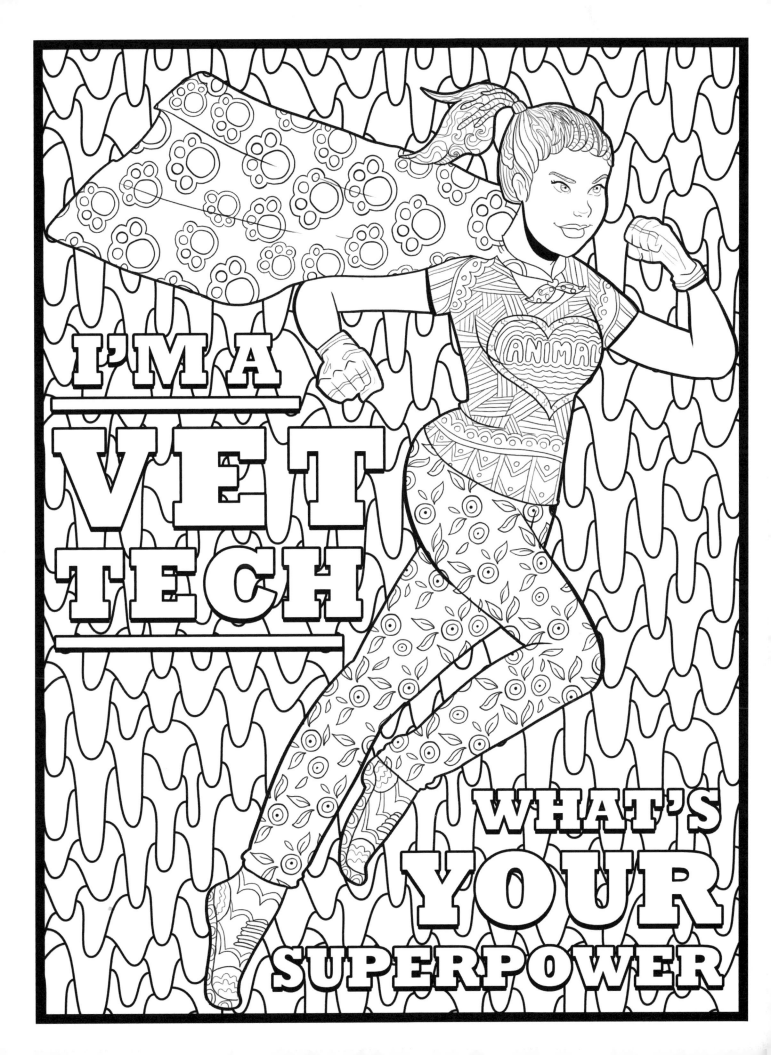

You know You're a VET TECH

WHEN ALL YOUR PETS ARE BLIND, 3-LEGGED, OR HAVE RARE MEDICAL CONDITIONS

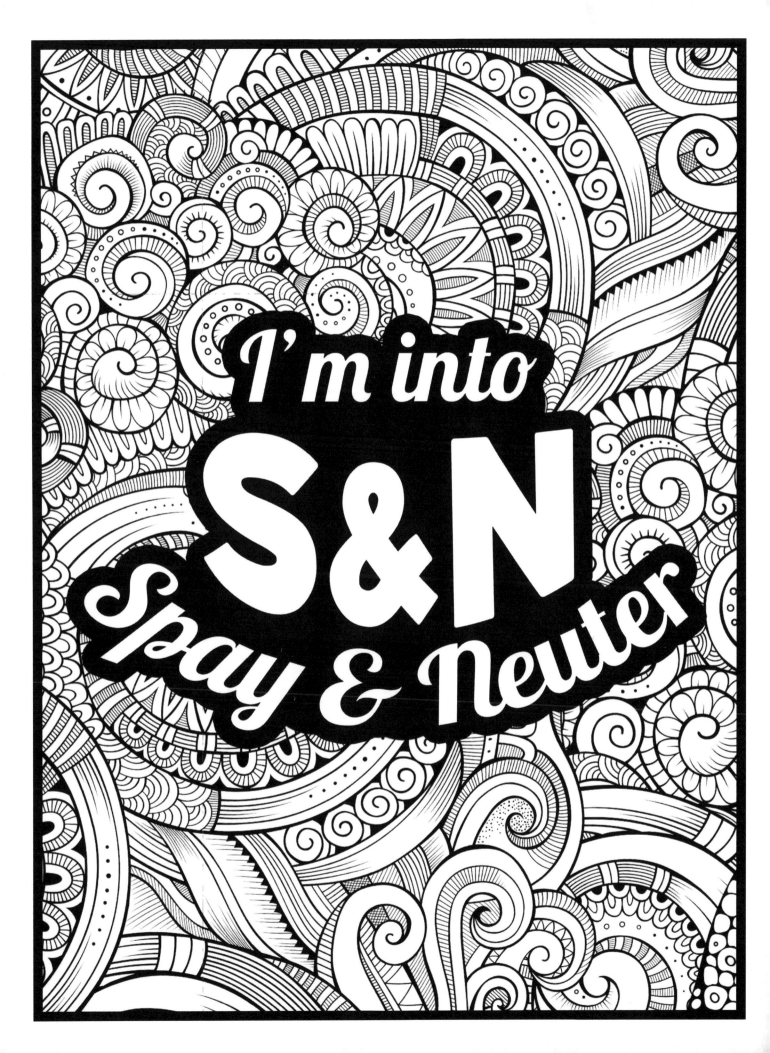

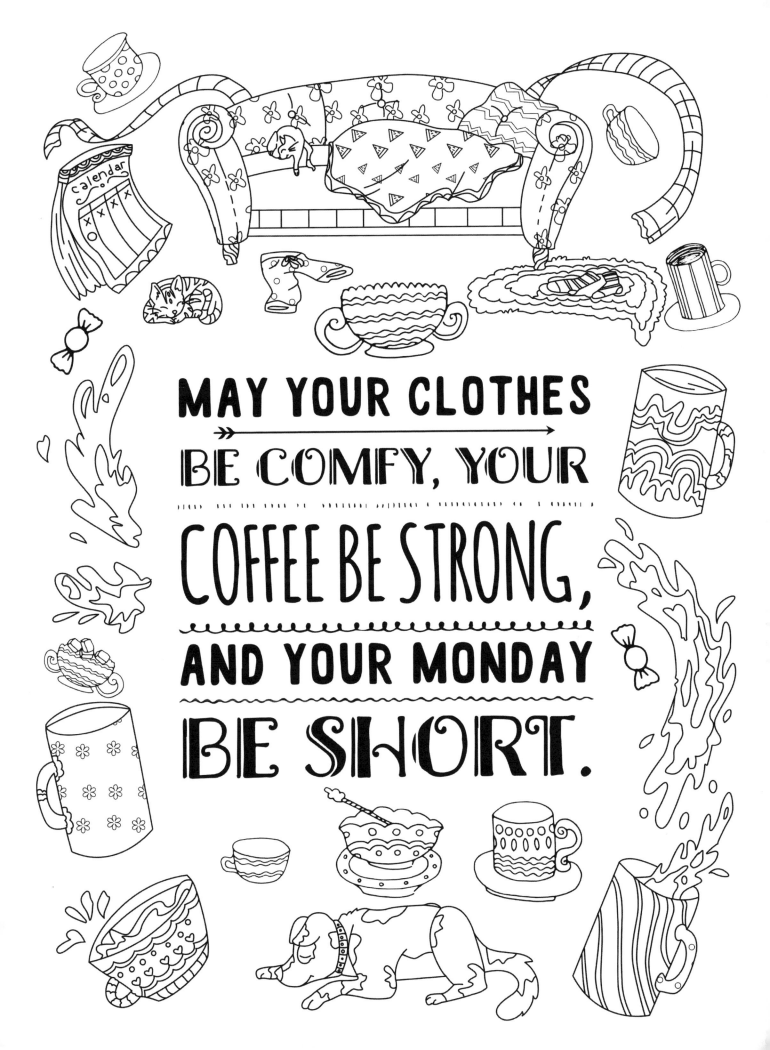

MAY YOUR CLOTHES BE COMFY, YOUR COFFEE BE STRONG, AND YOUR MONDAY BE SHORT.

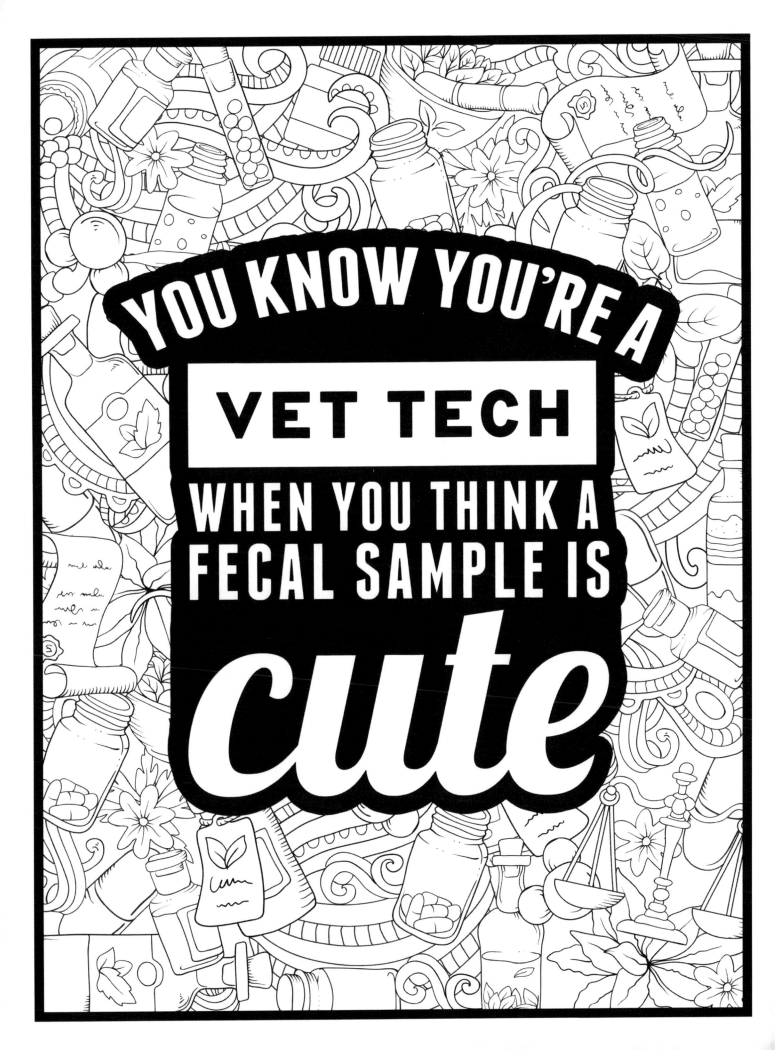

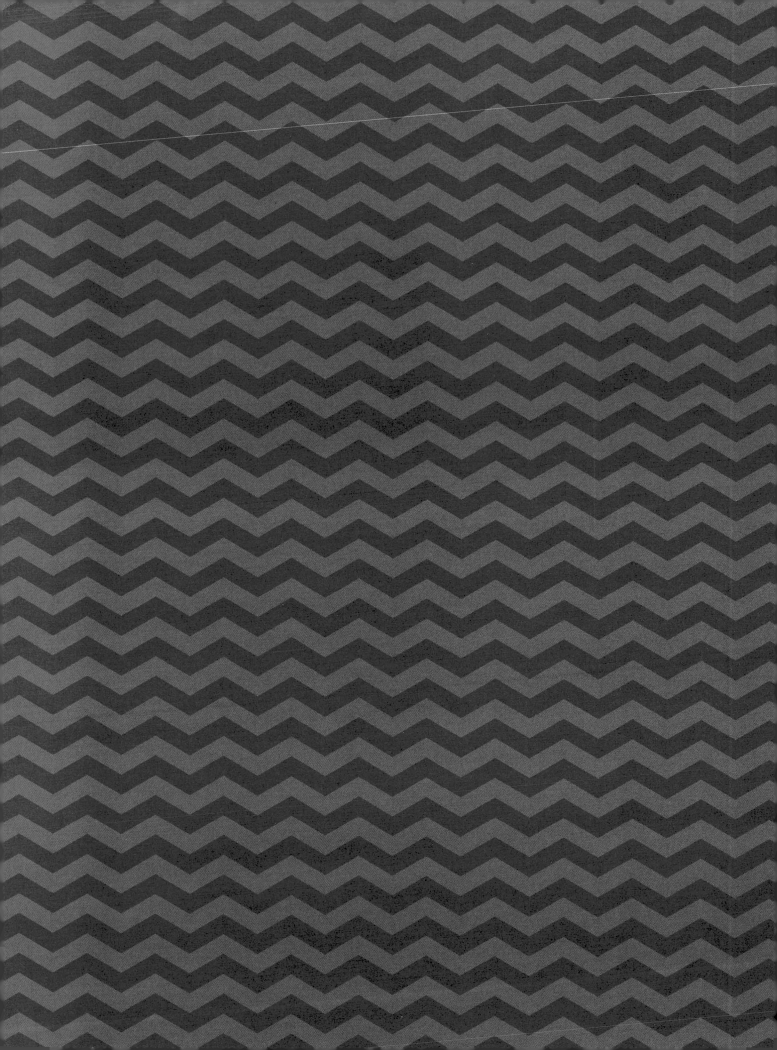

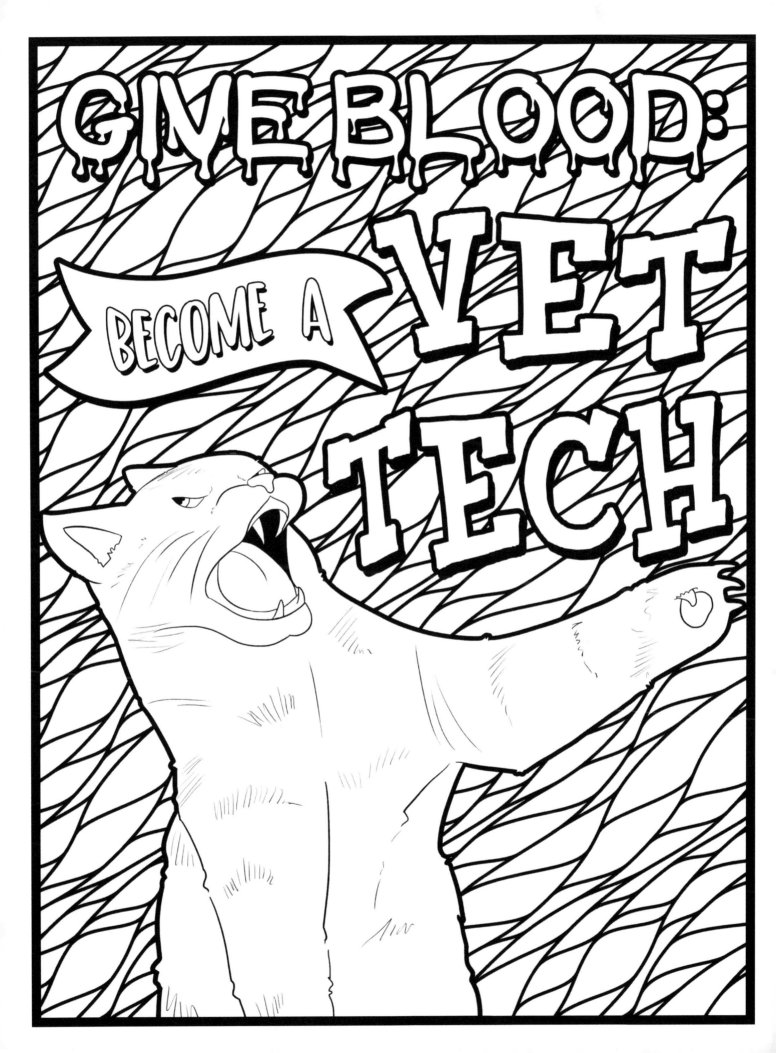

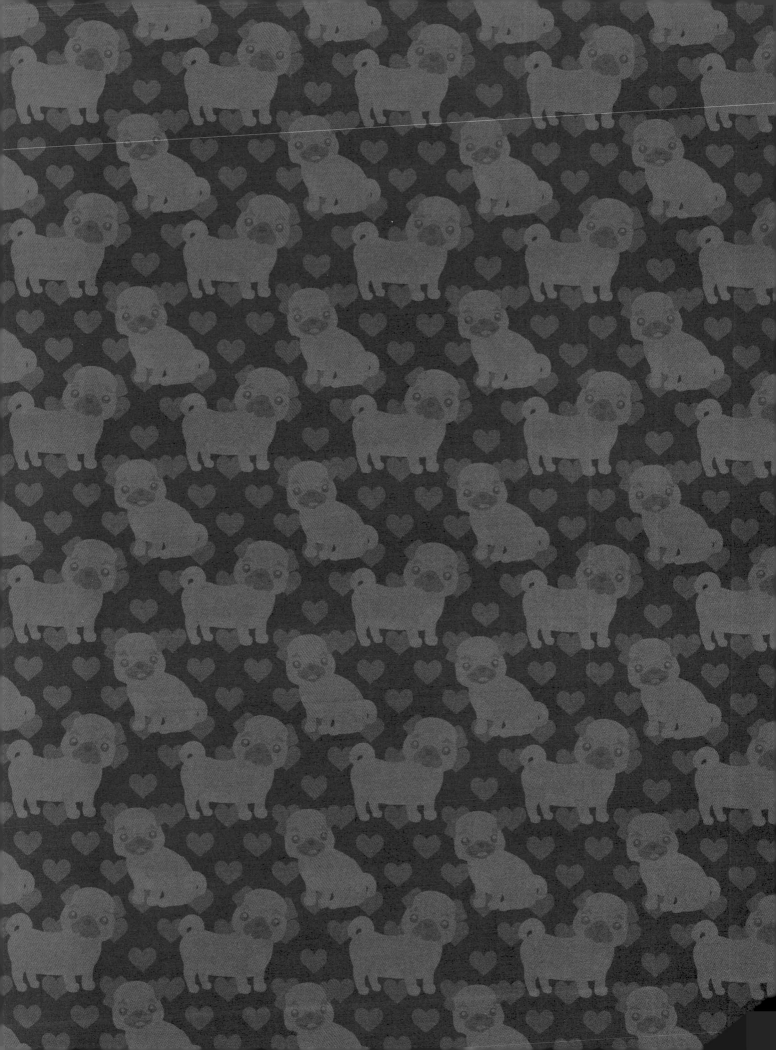

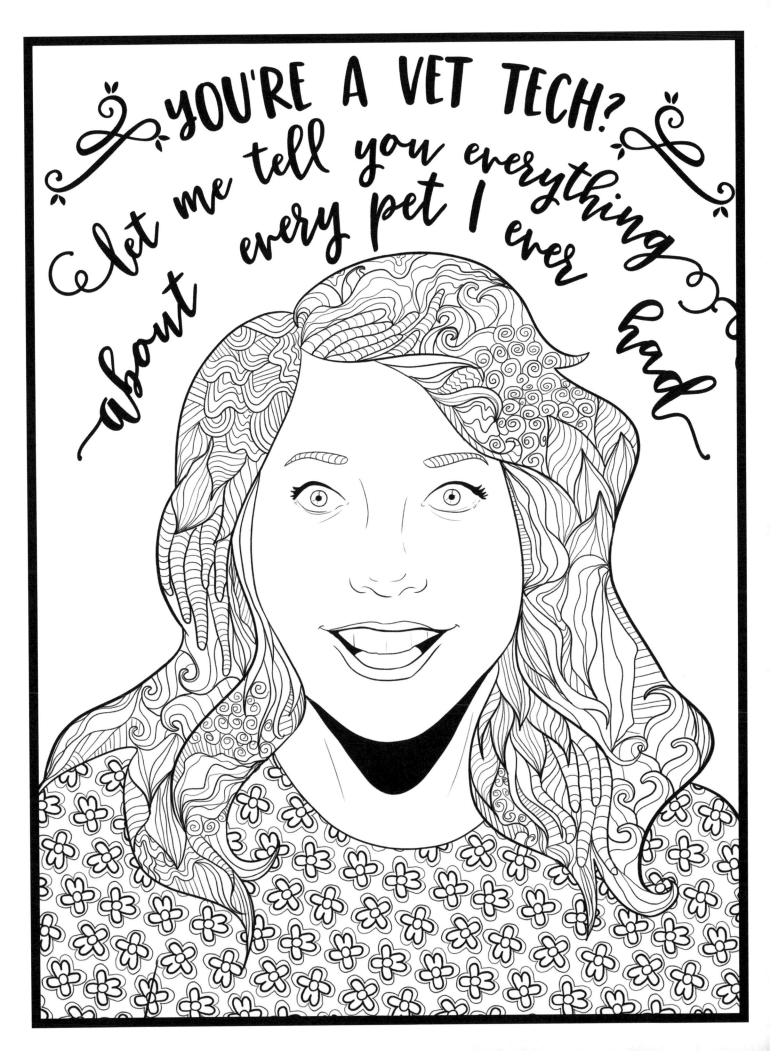

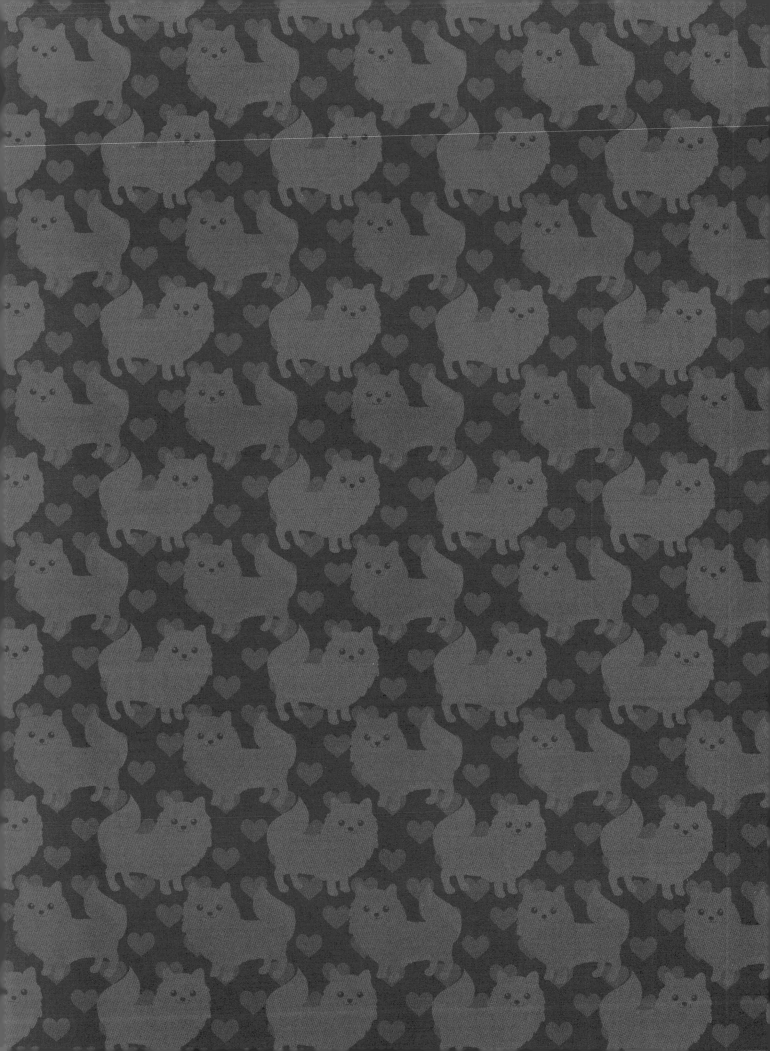

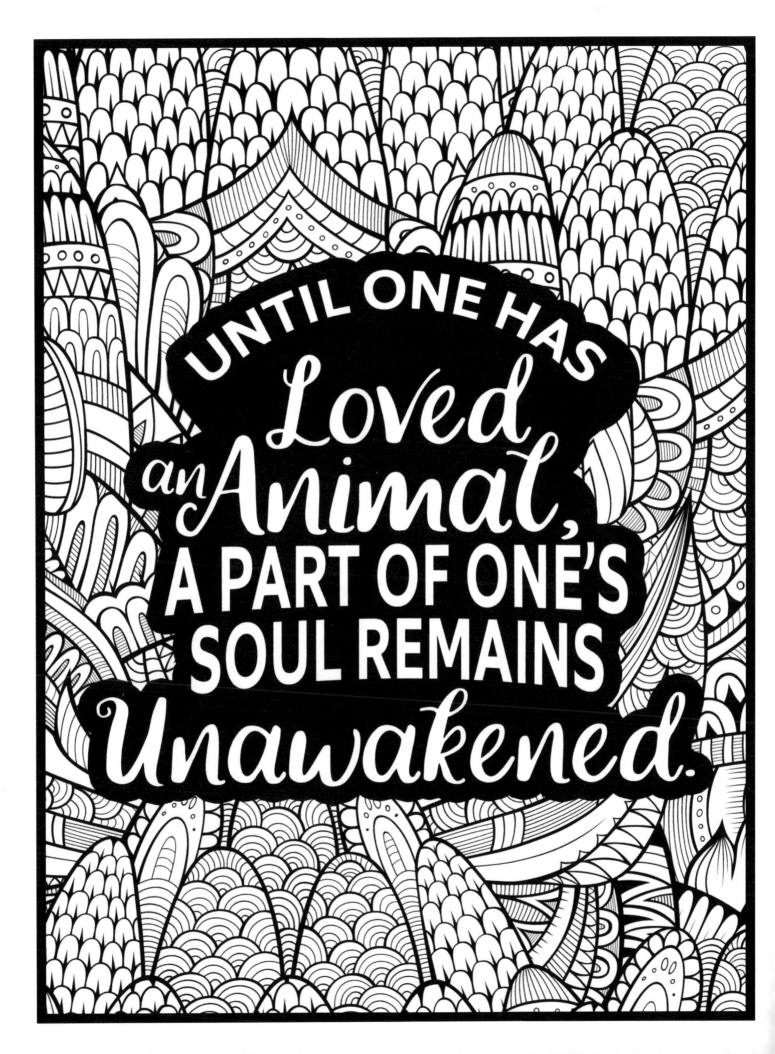

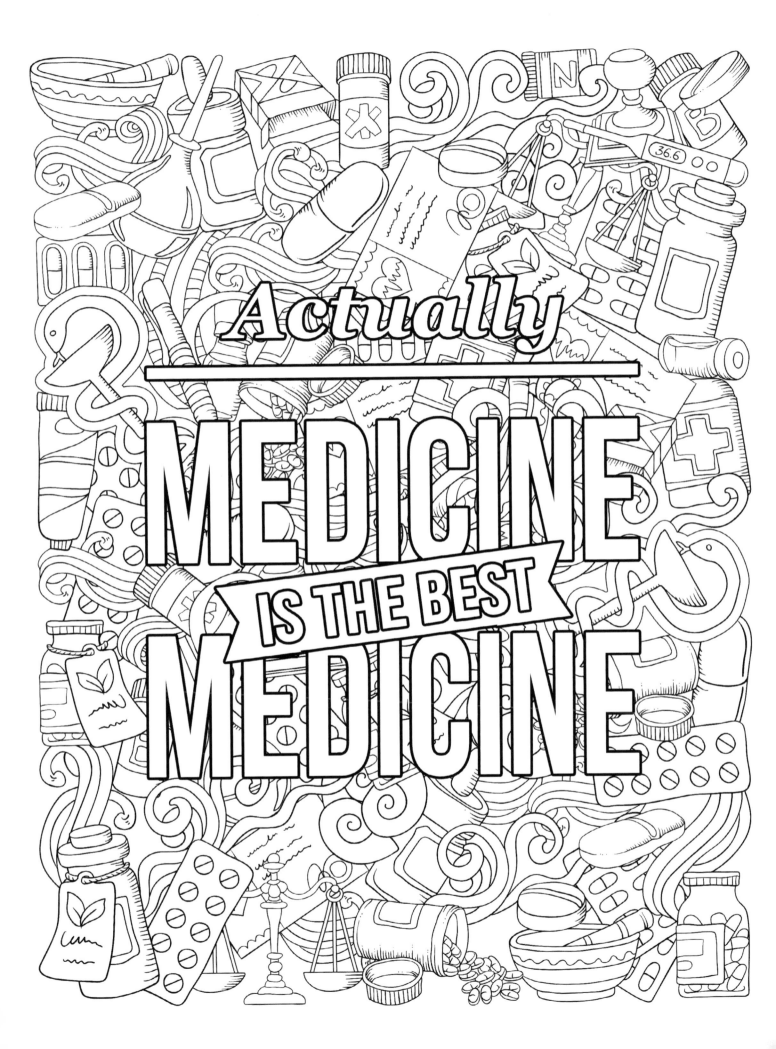

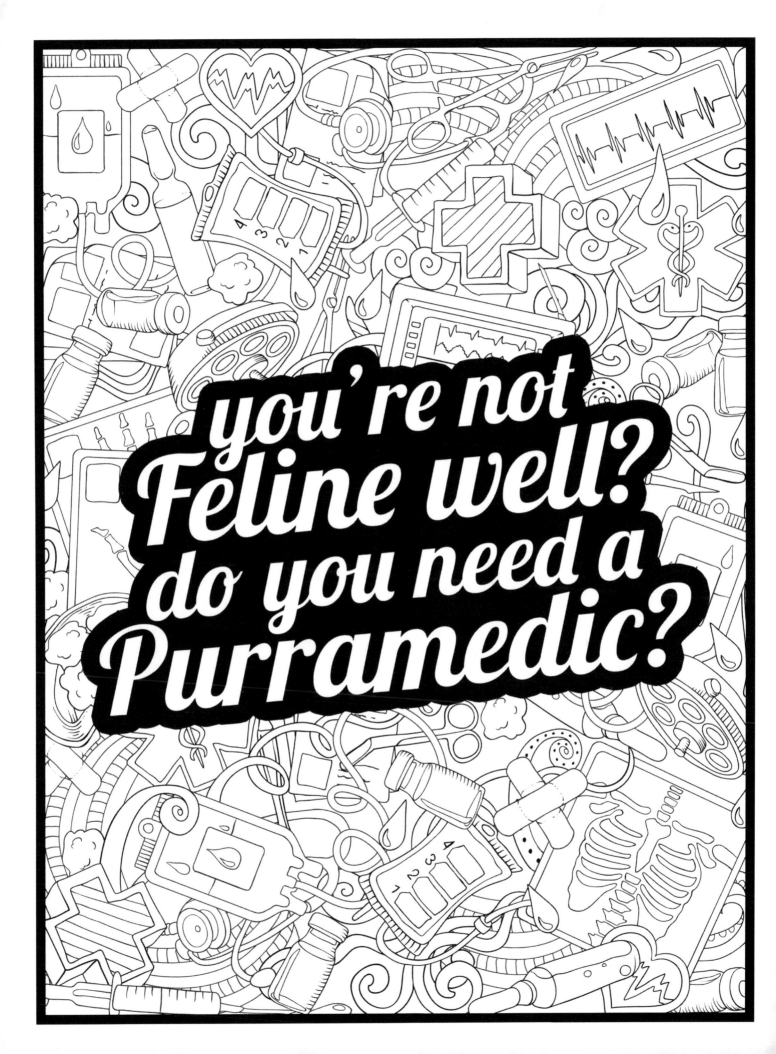

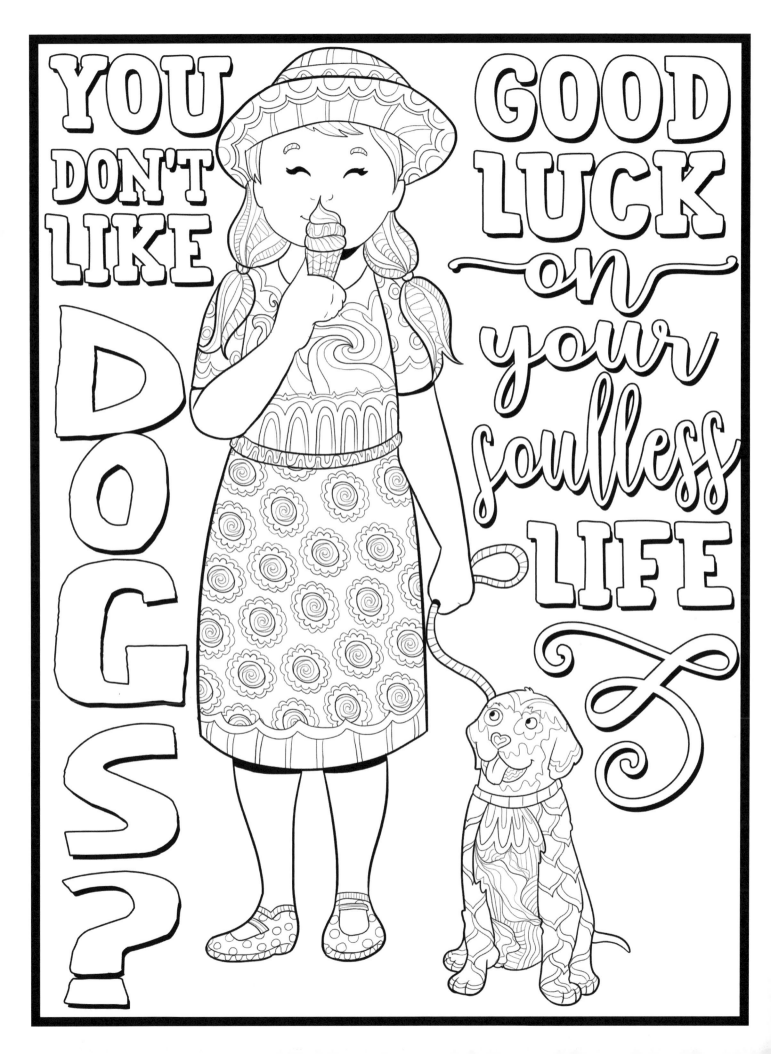

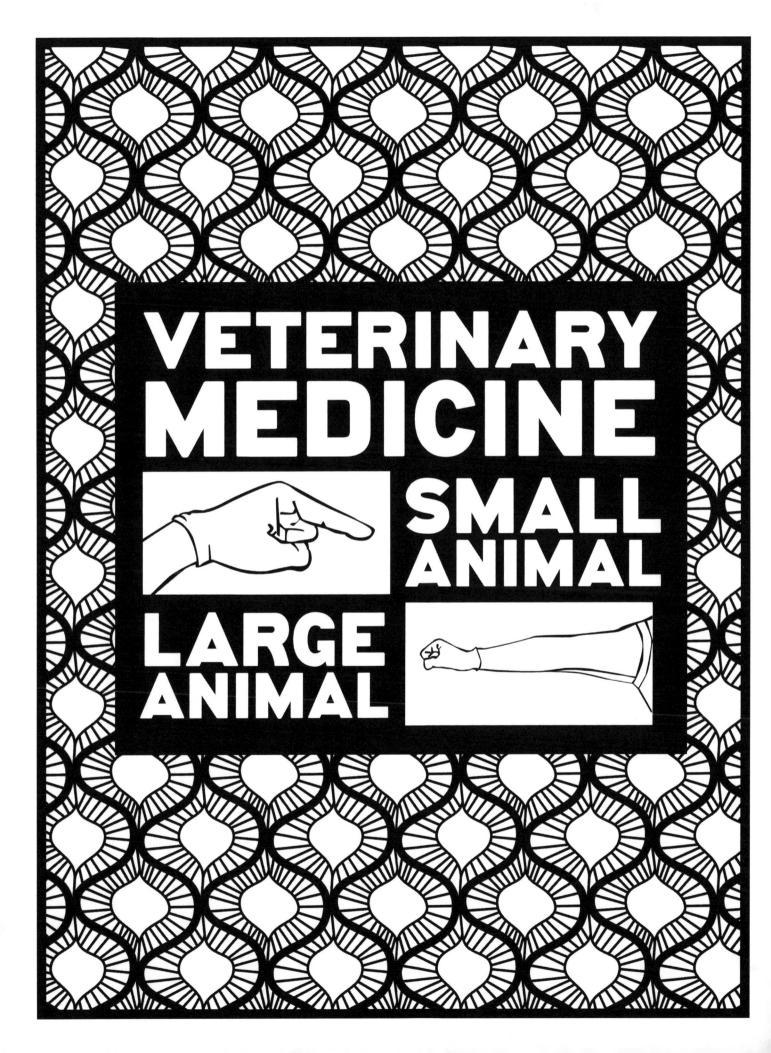

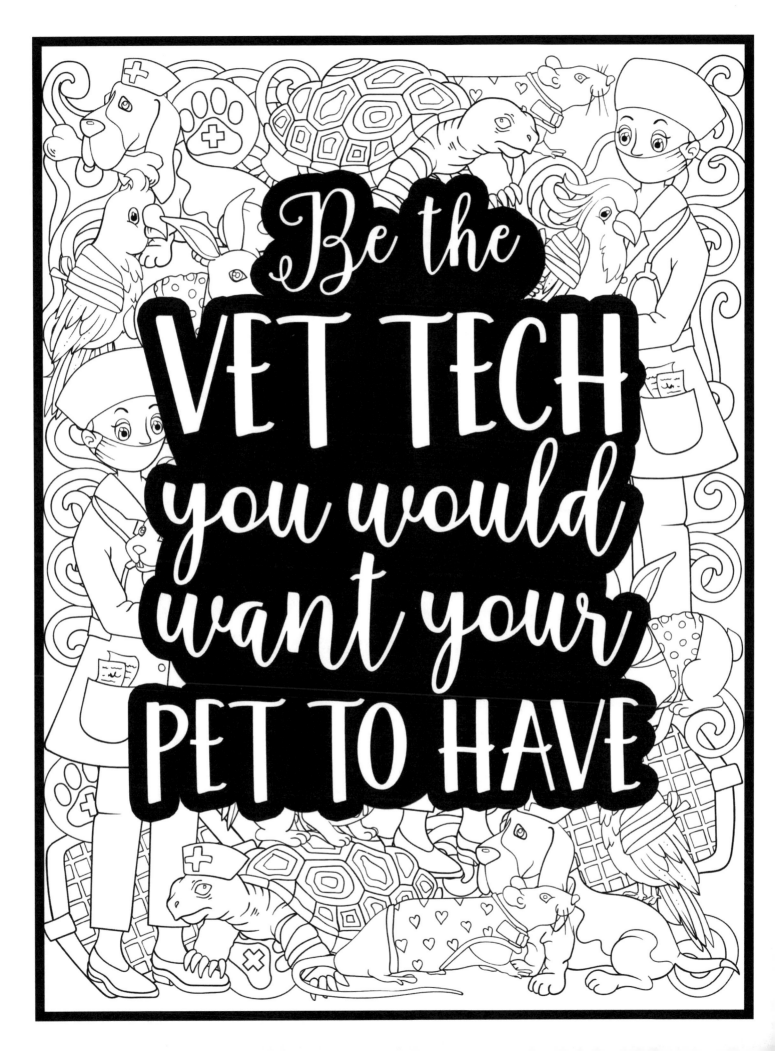

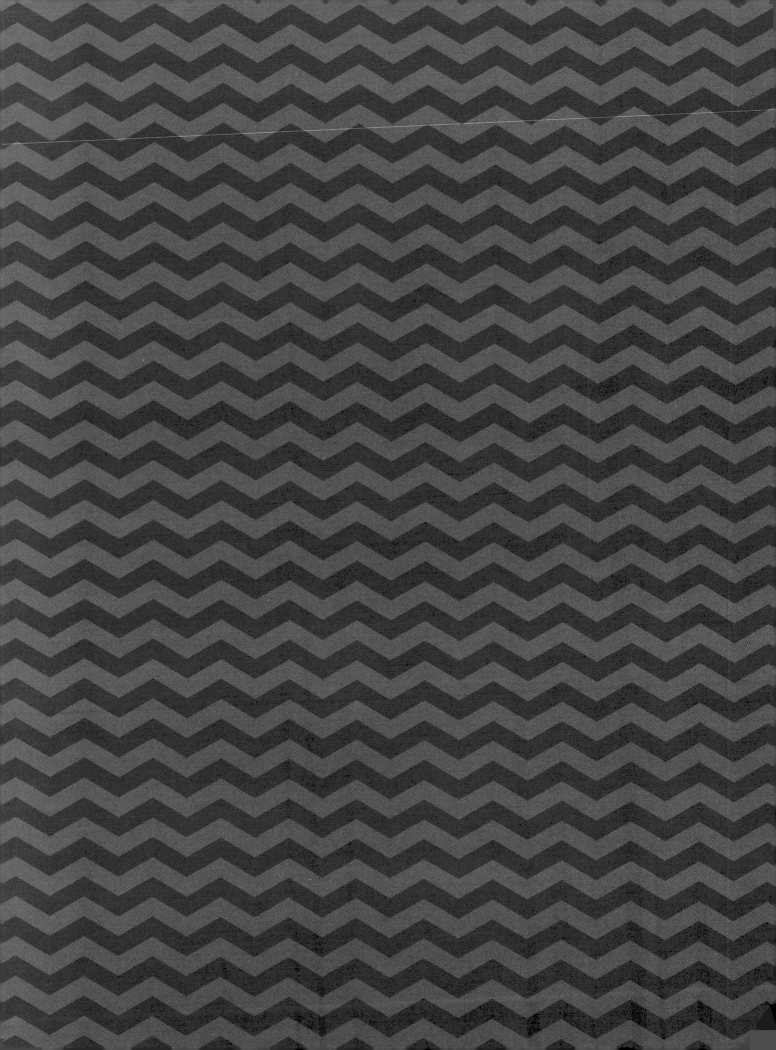

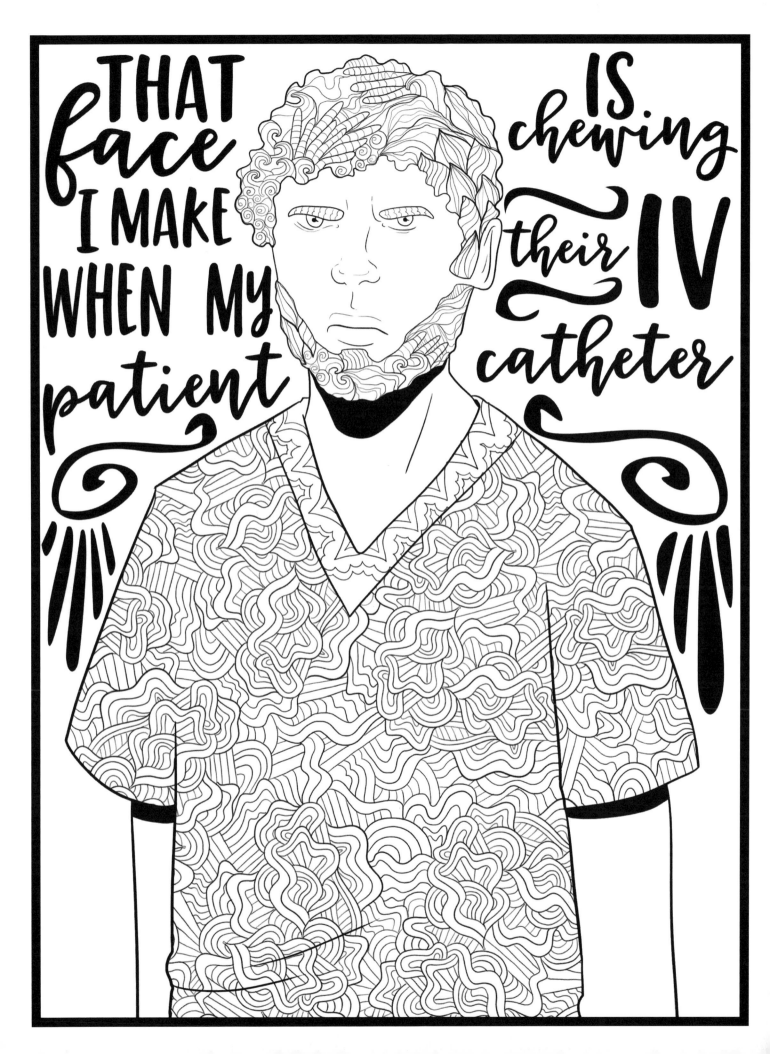

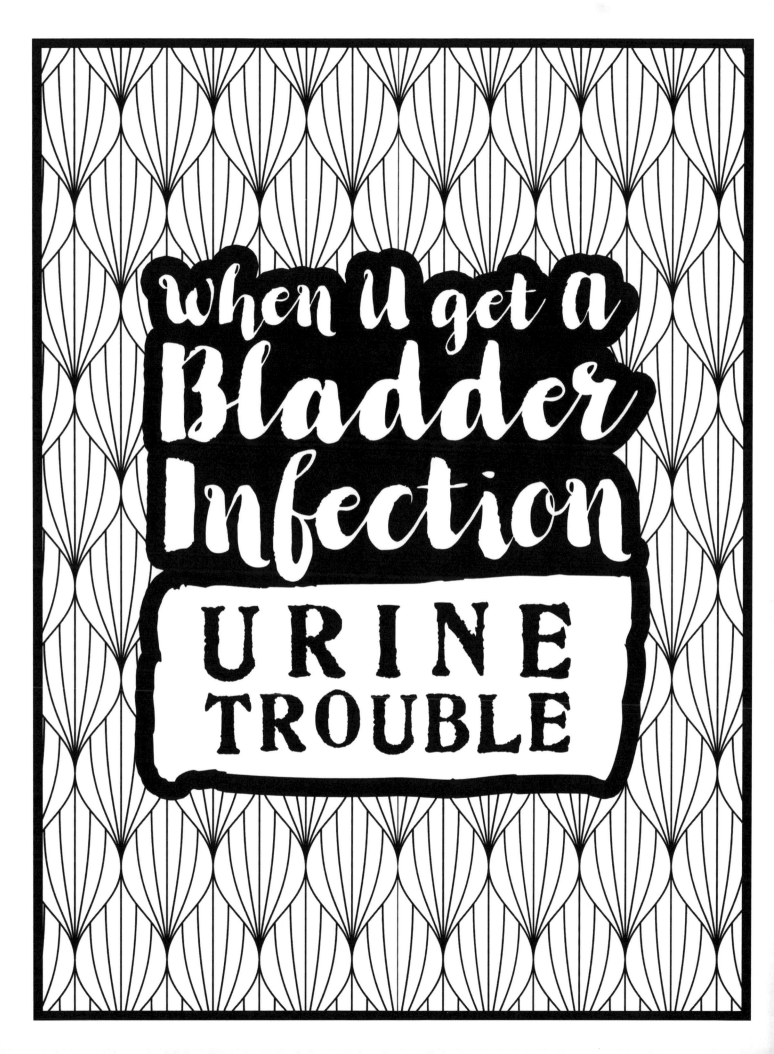

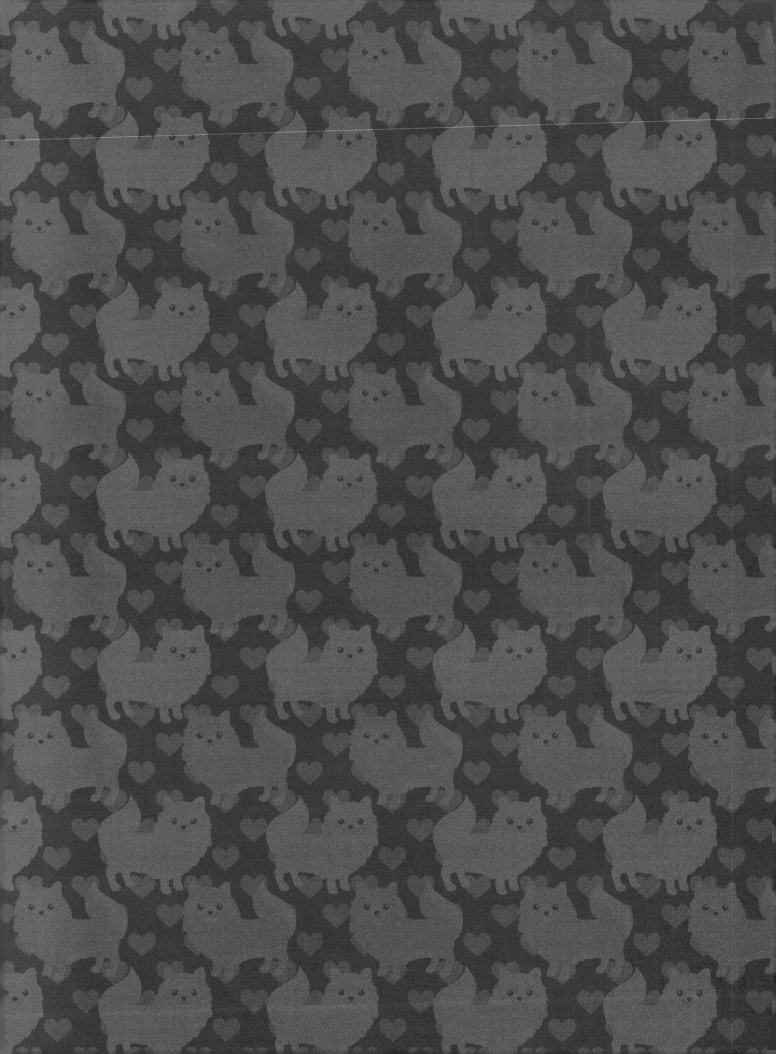

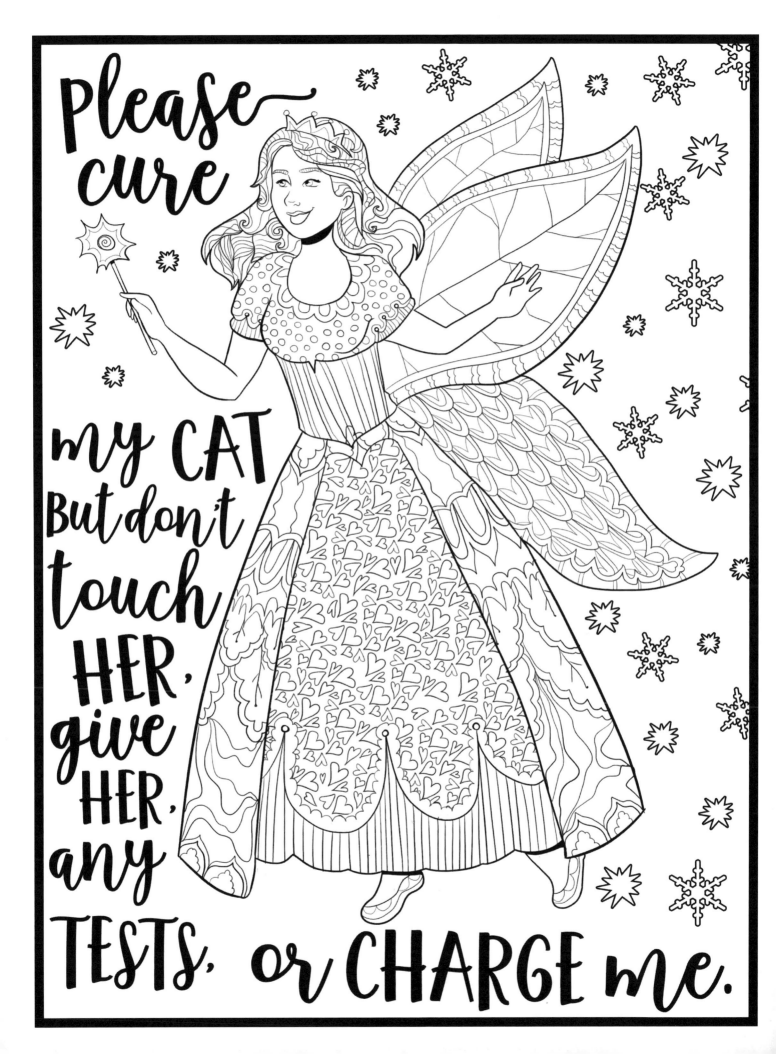

Please cure my CAT But don't touch HER, give HER, any TESTS, or CHARGE me.

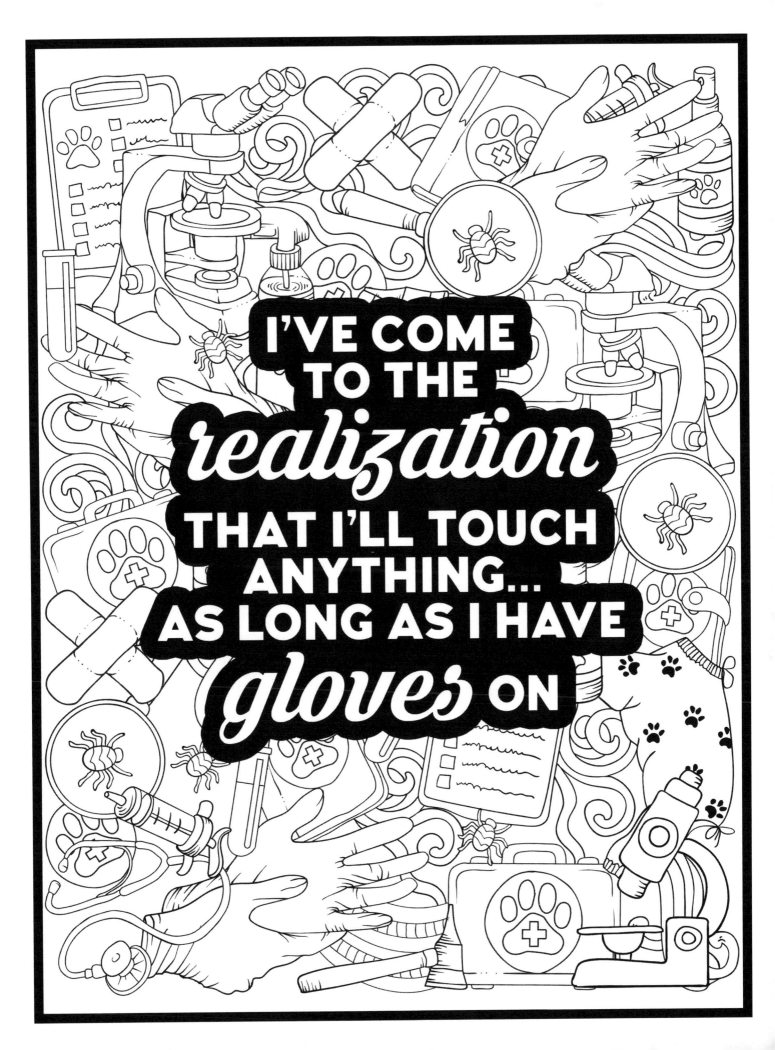

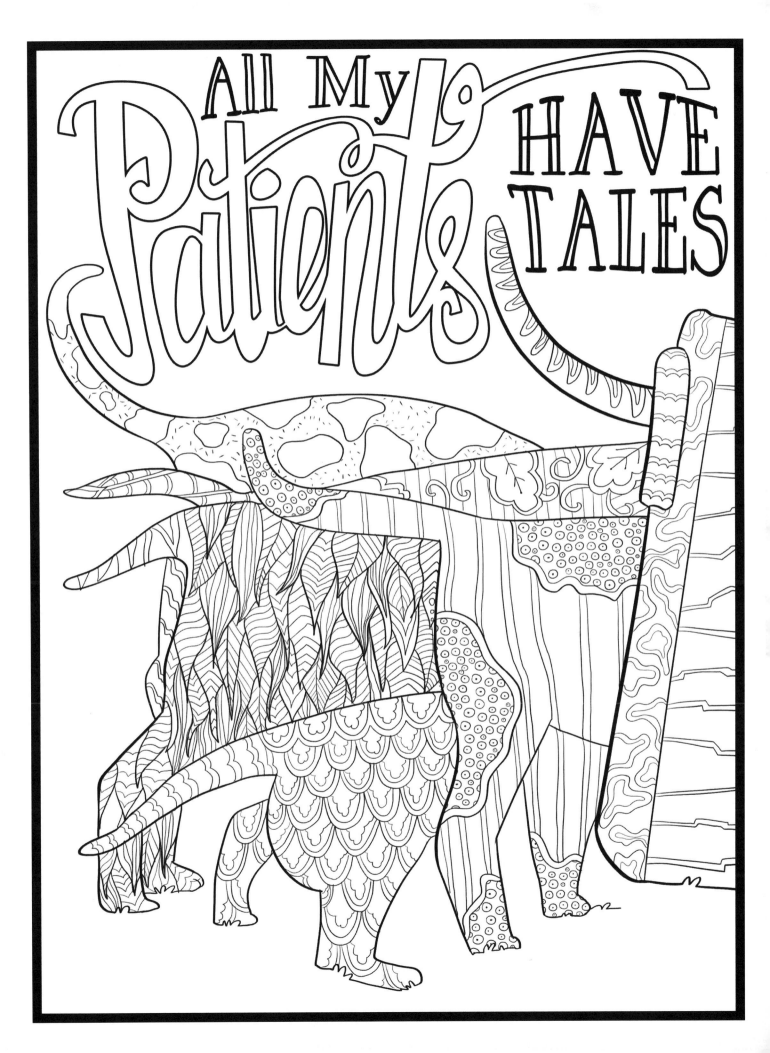

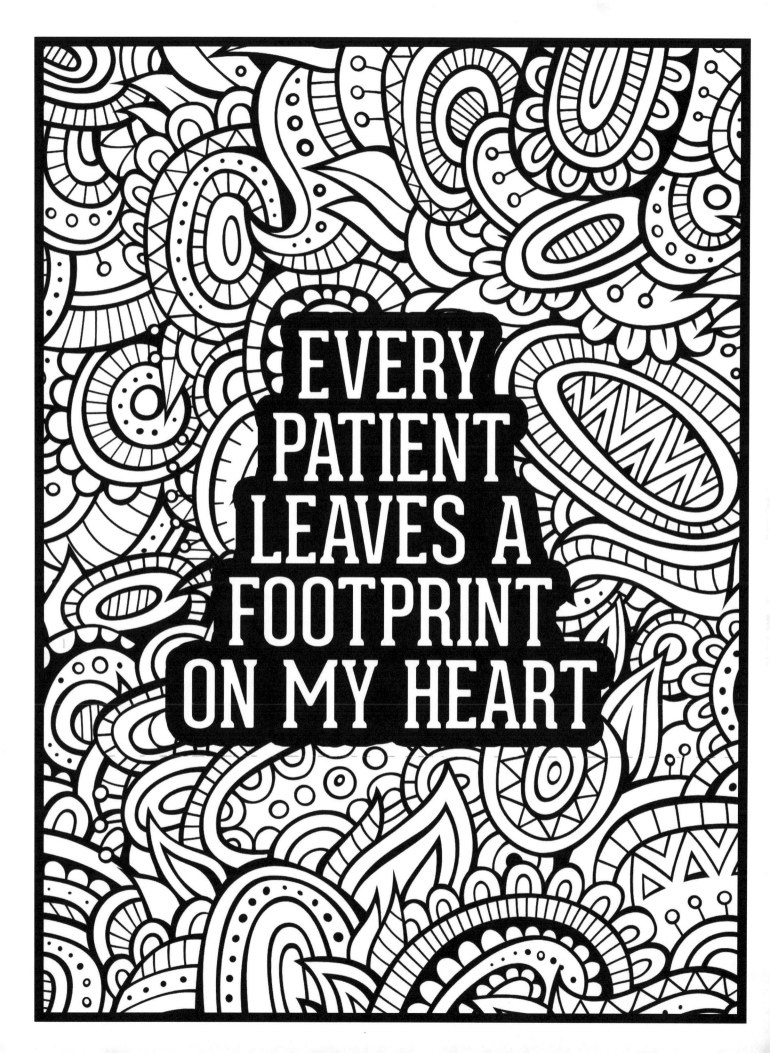

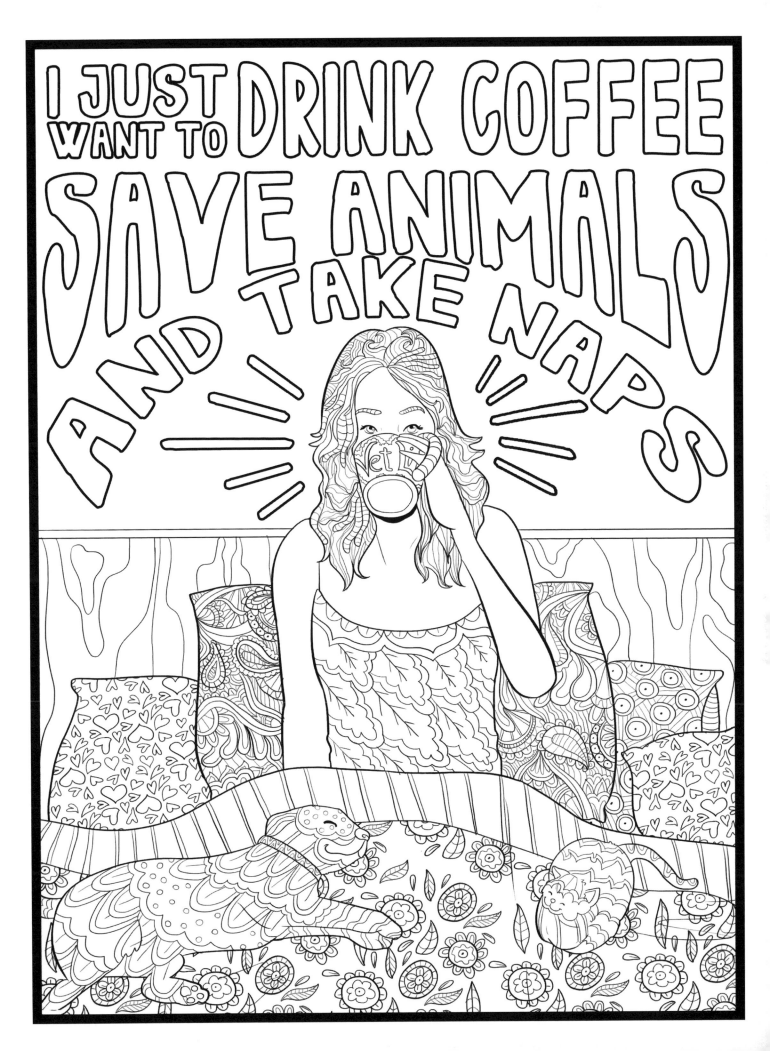

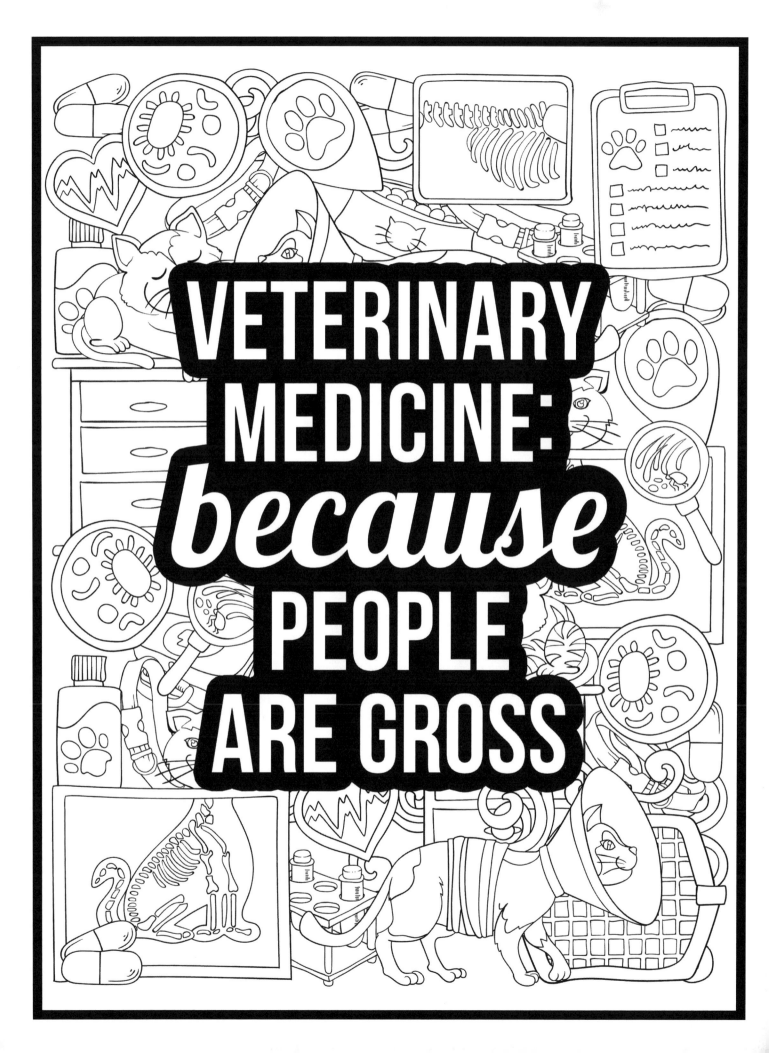

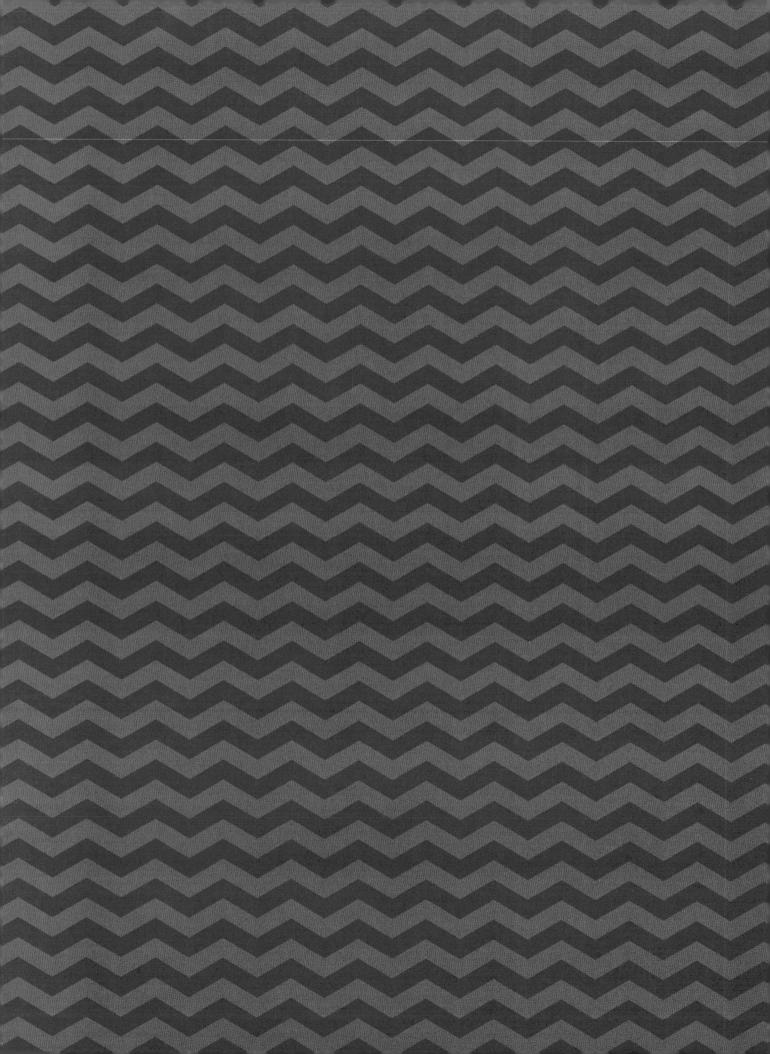

MY JUDGMENTAL VET TECH FACE WHEN SOMEONE REFUSES TO SPAY OR NEUTER THEIR PET

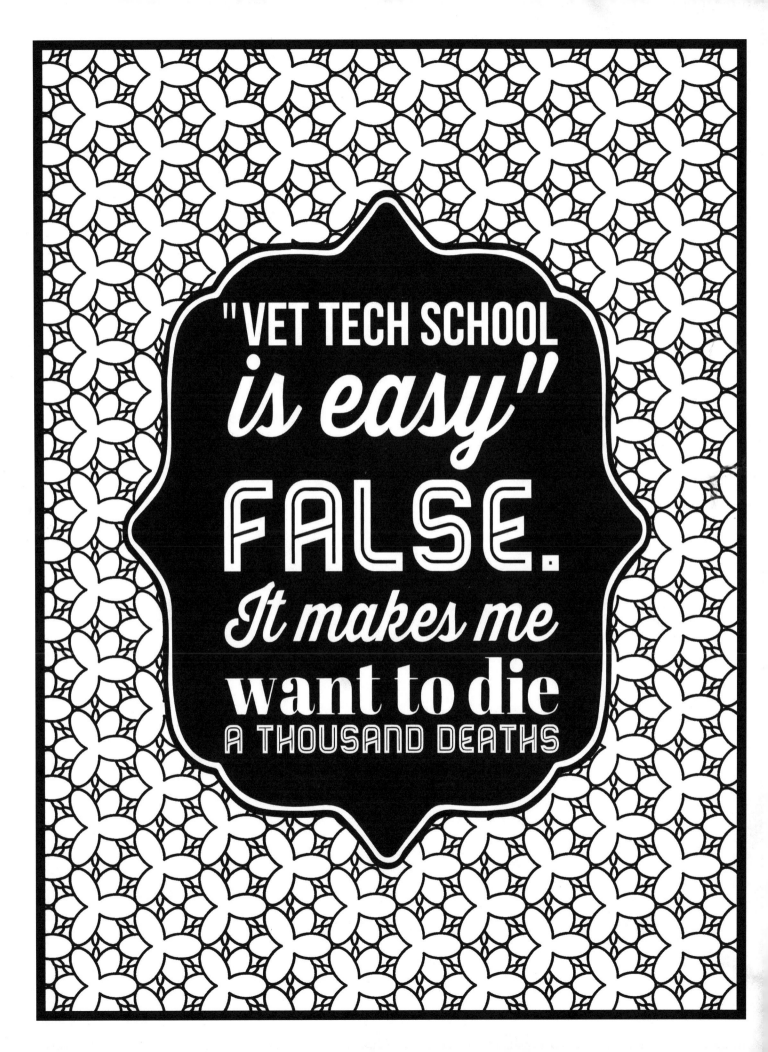

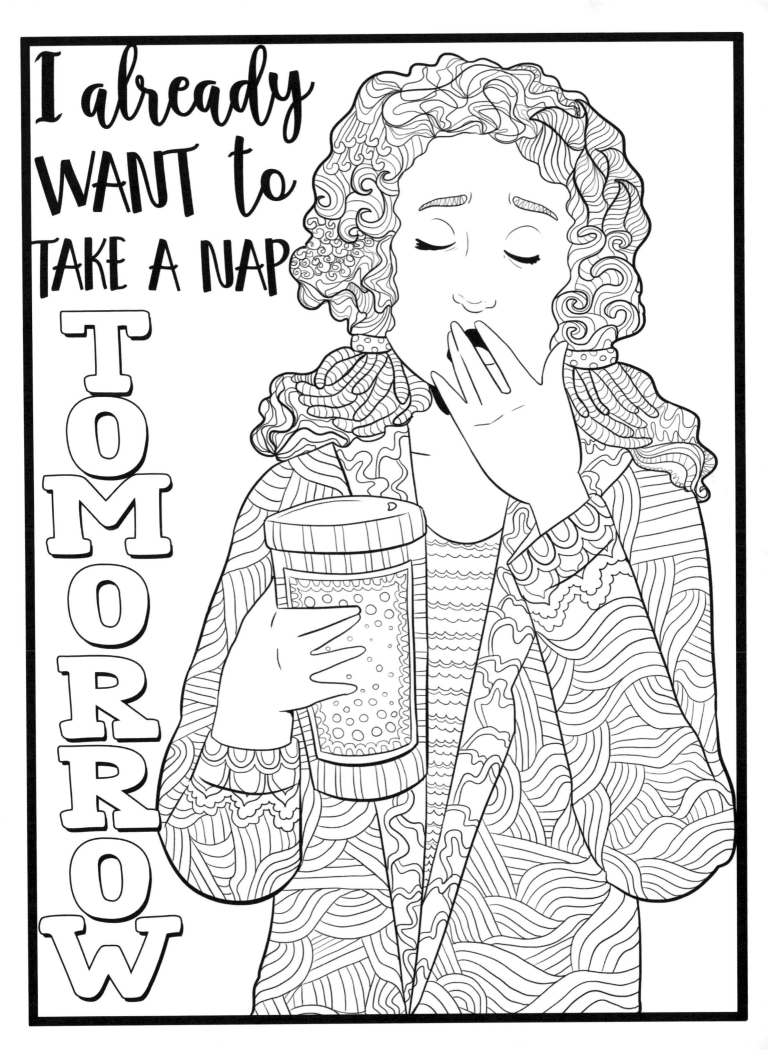

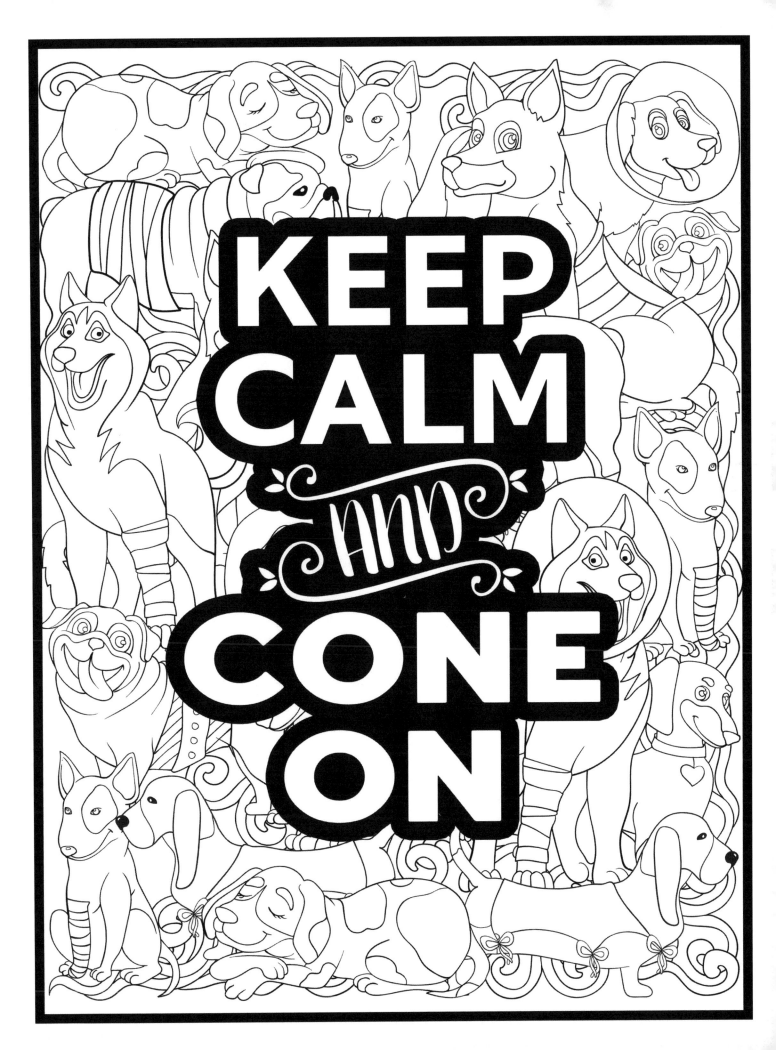

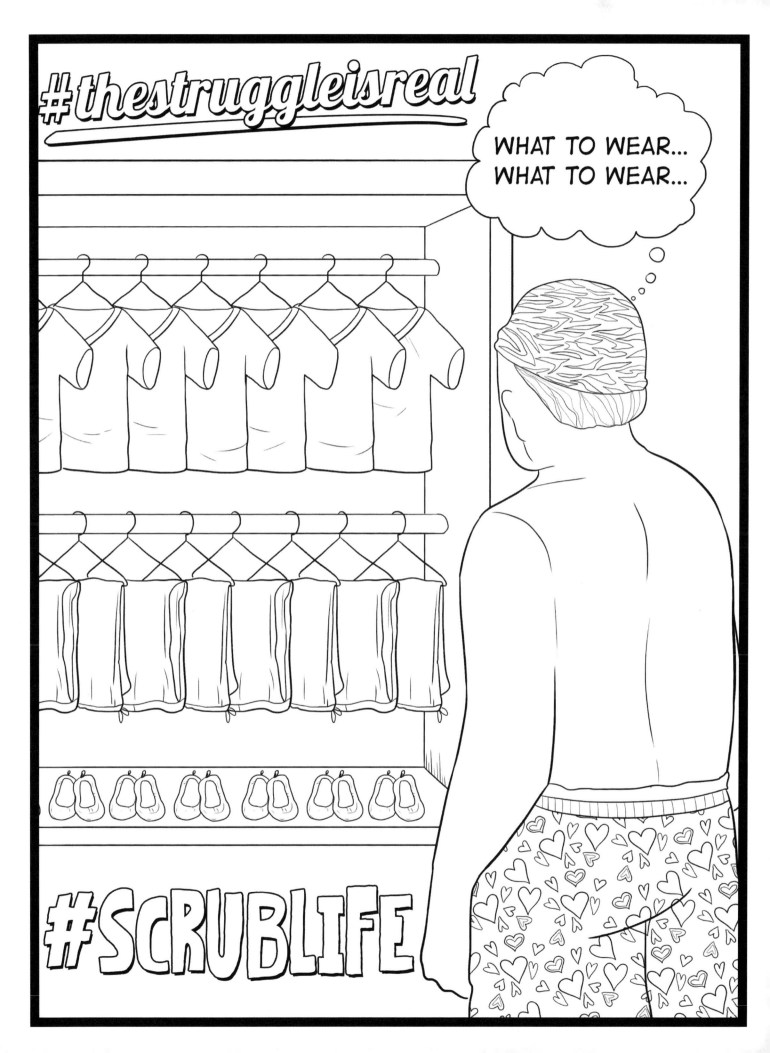

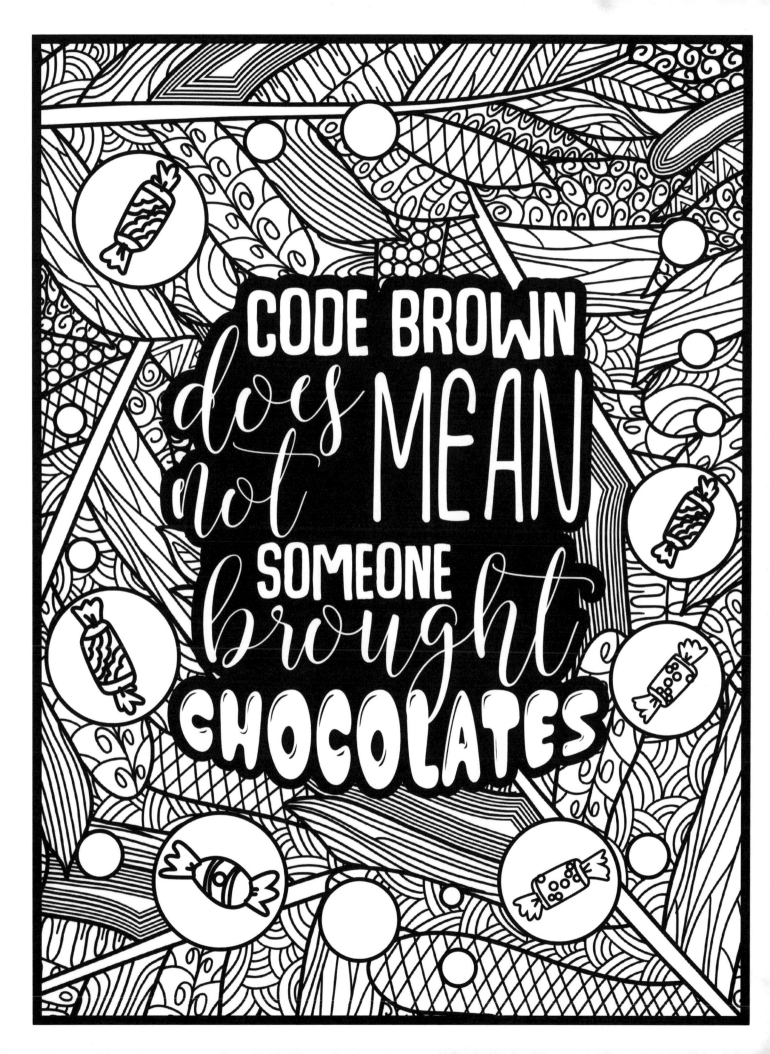

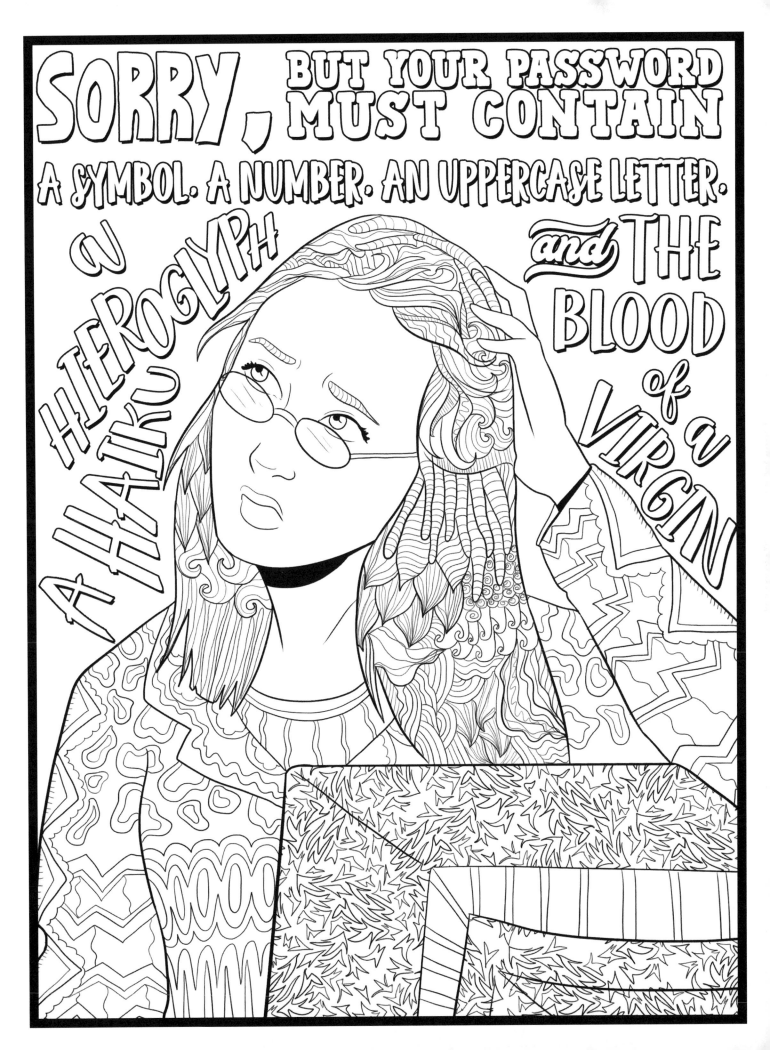

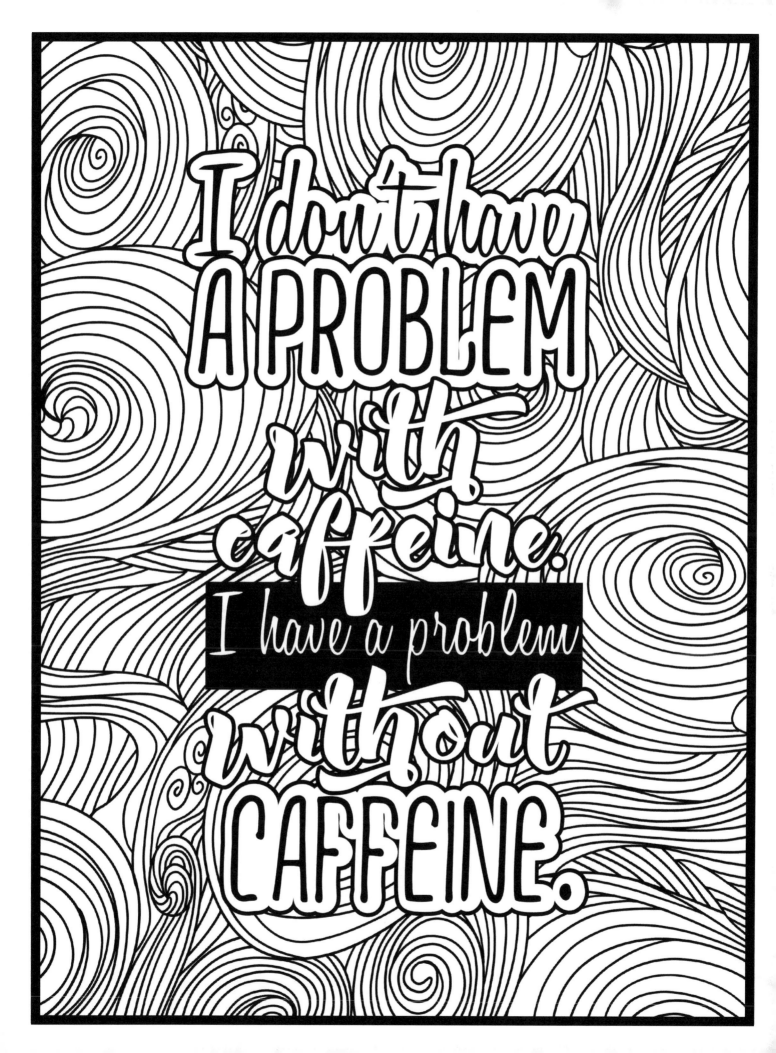

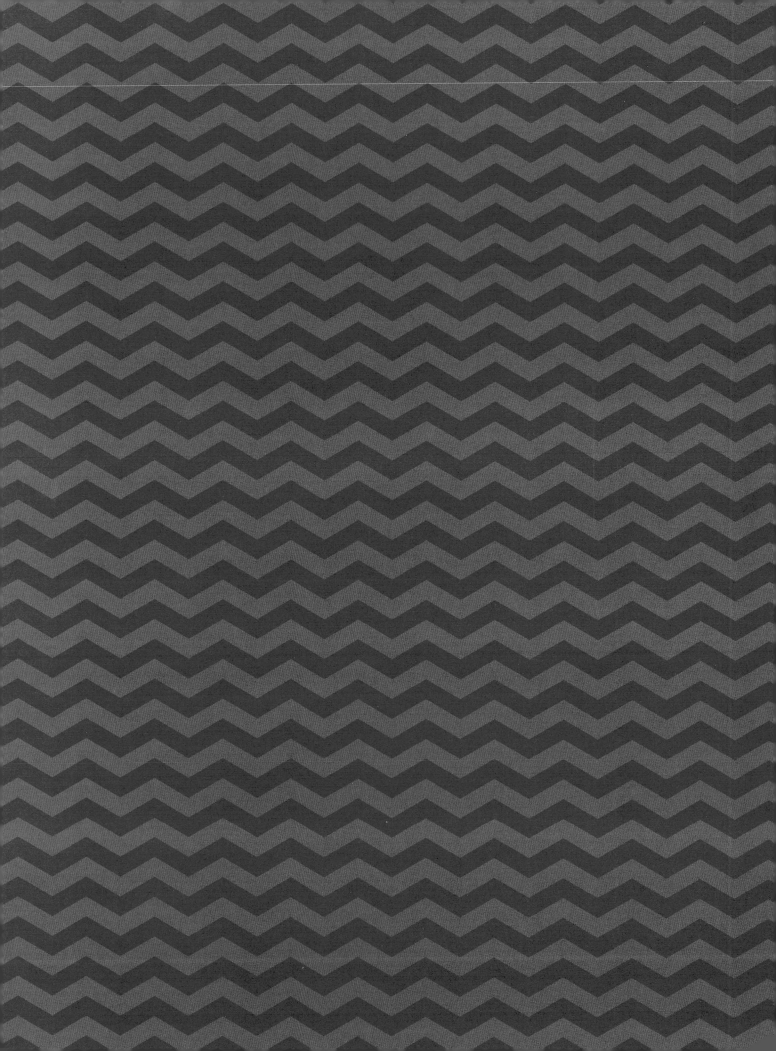

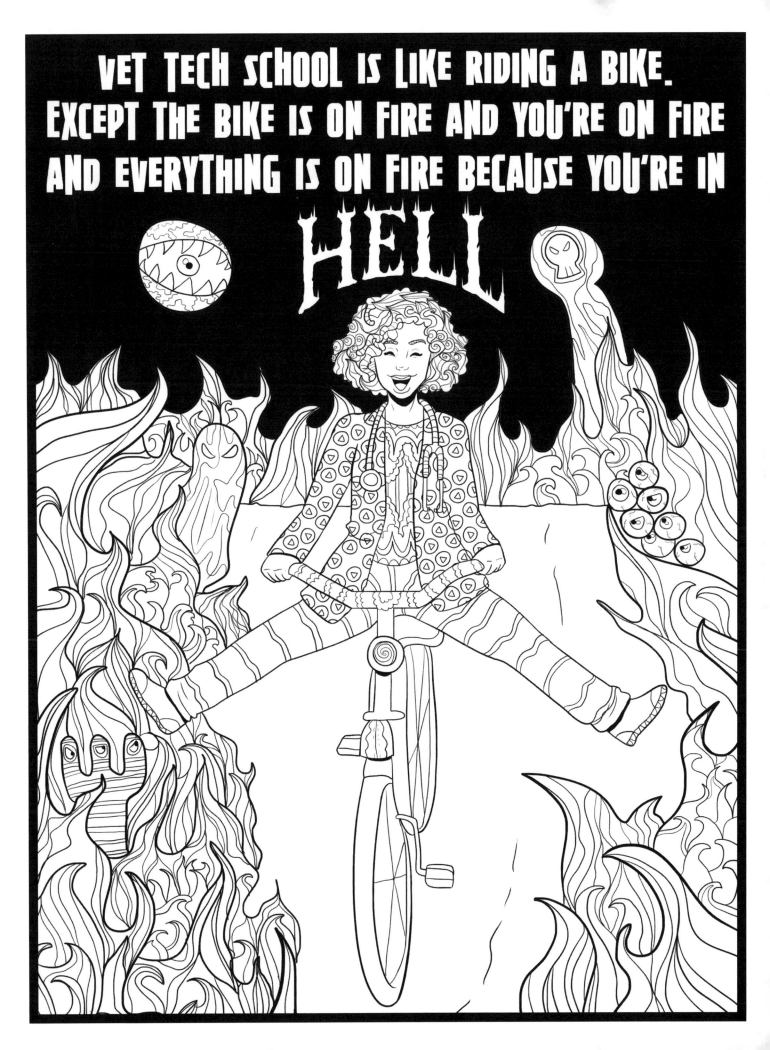

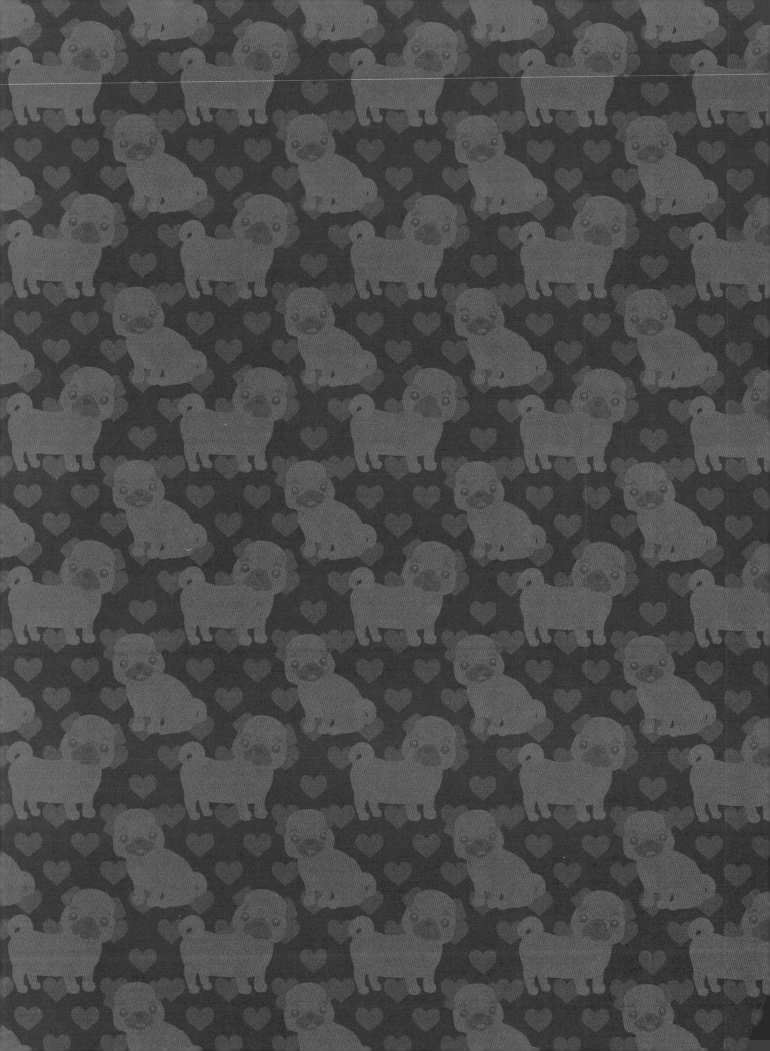

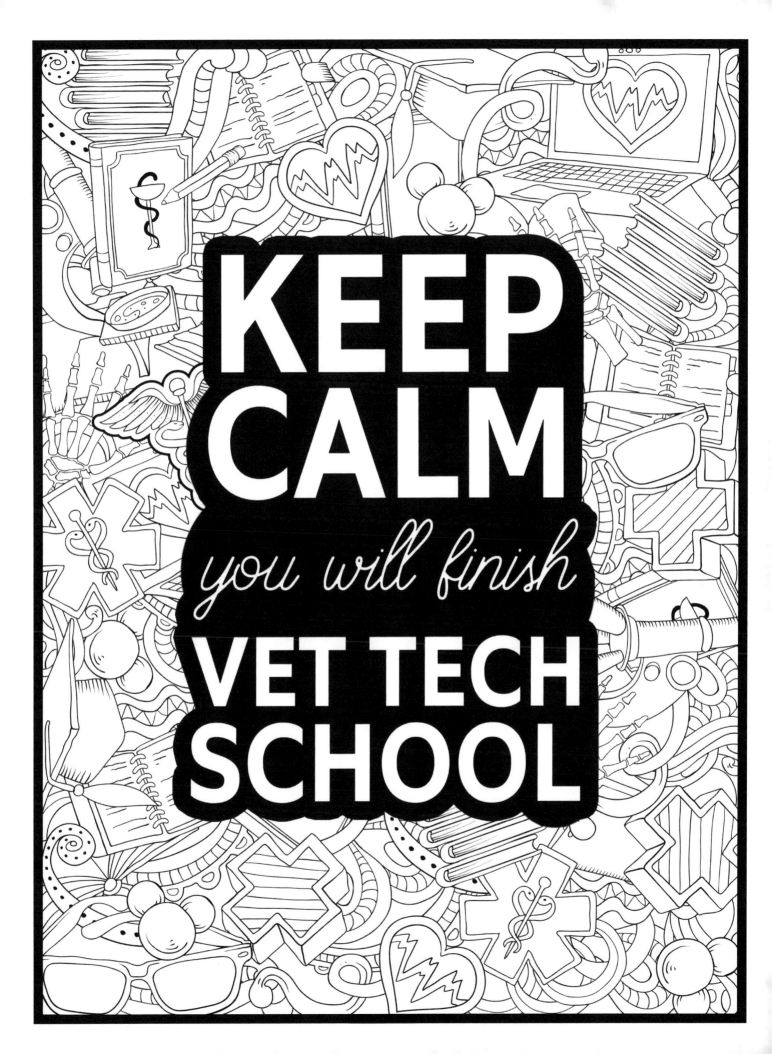

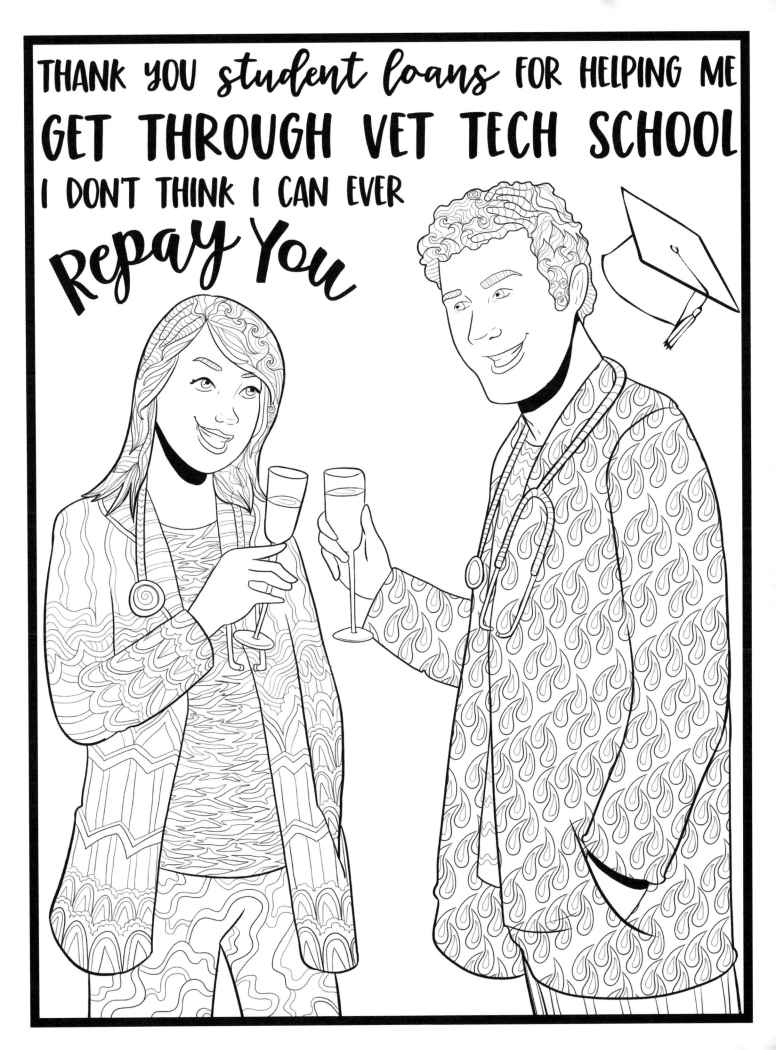

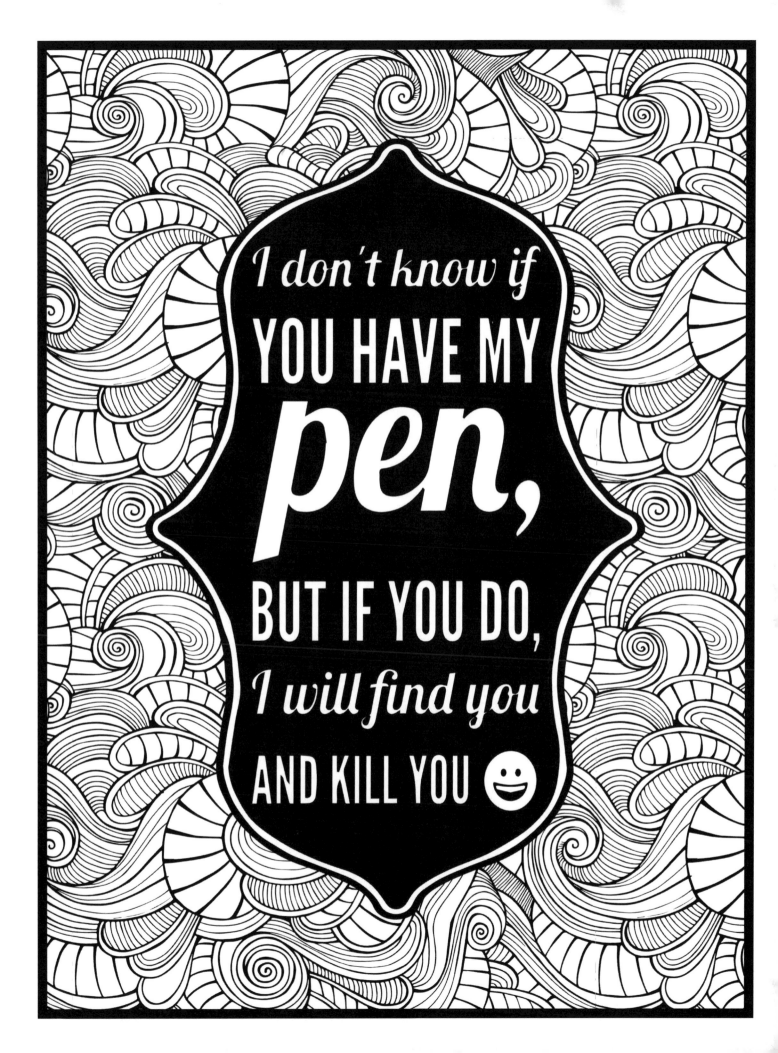

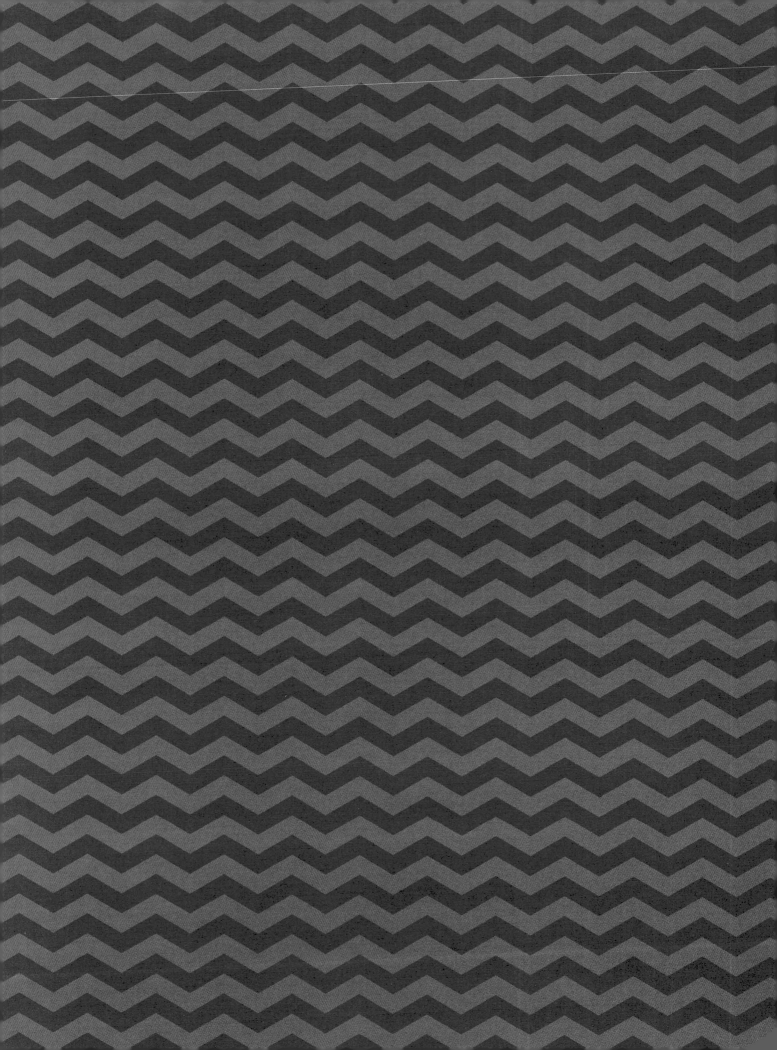

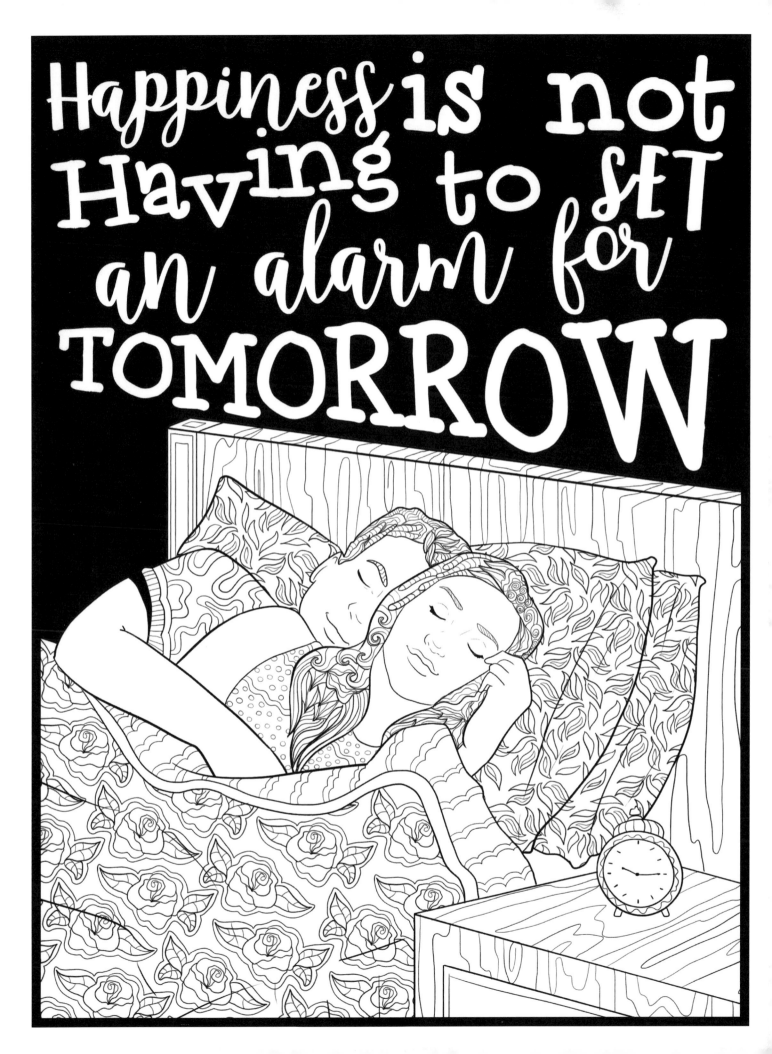

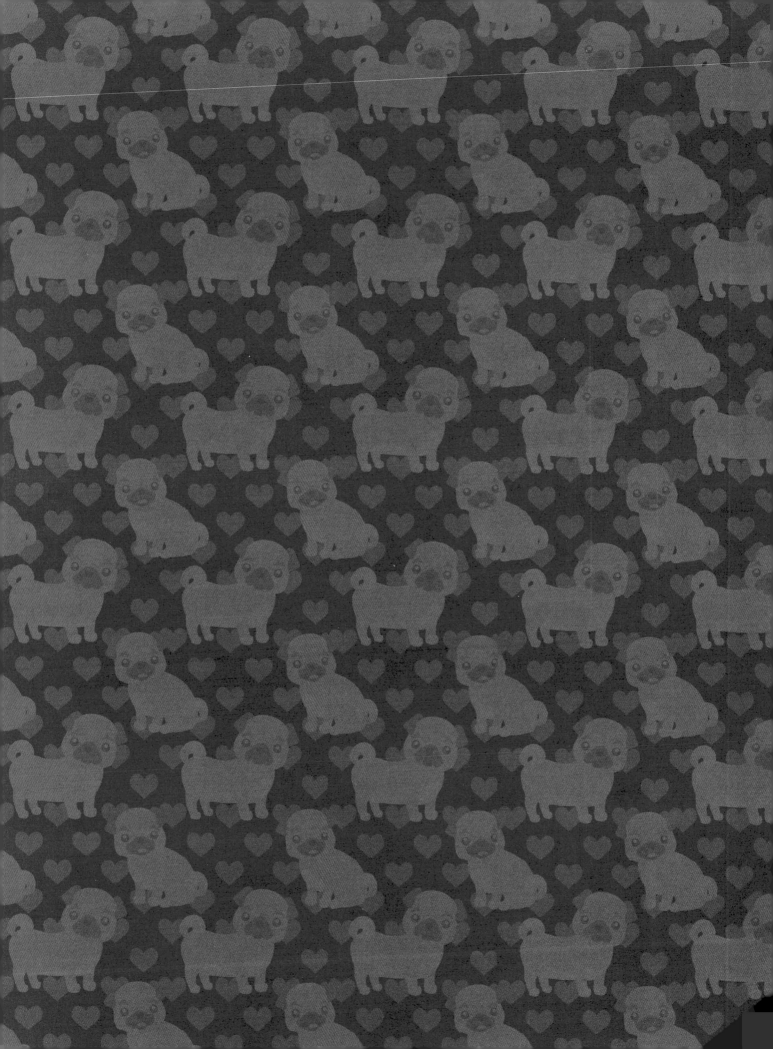

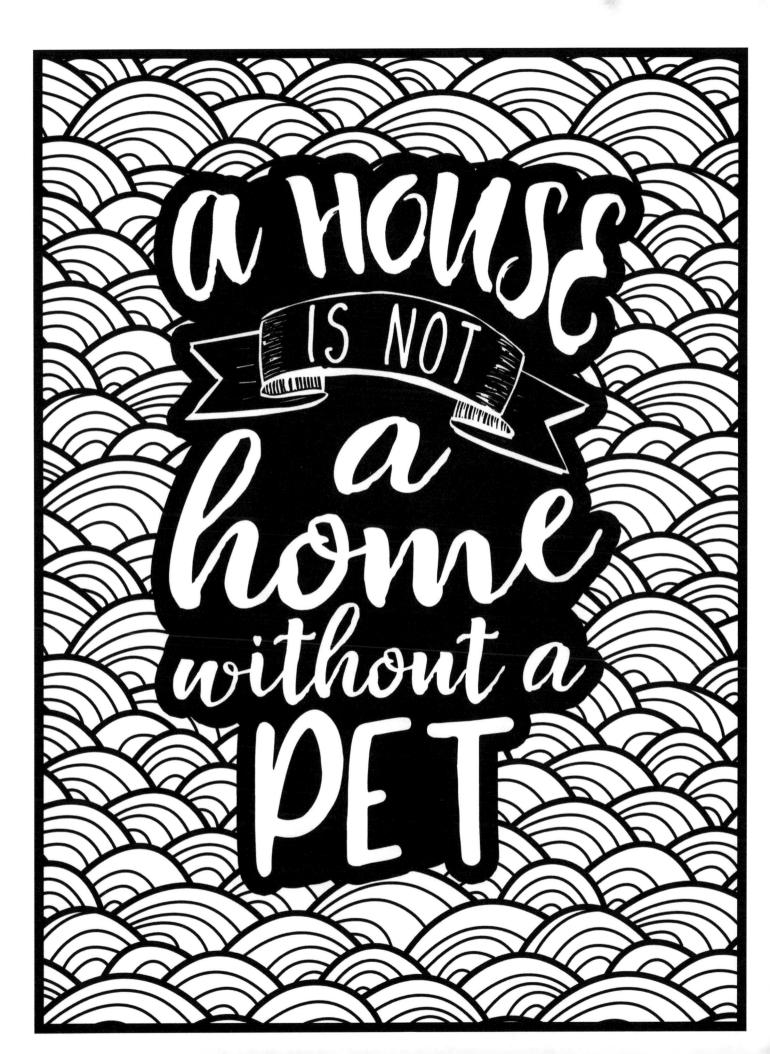

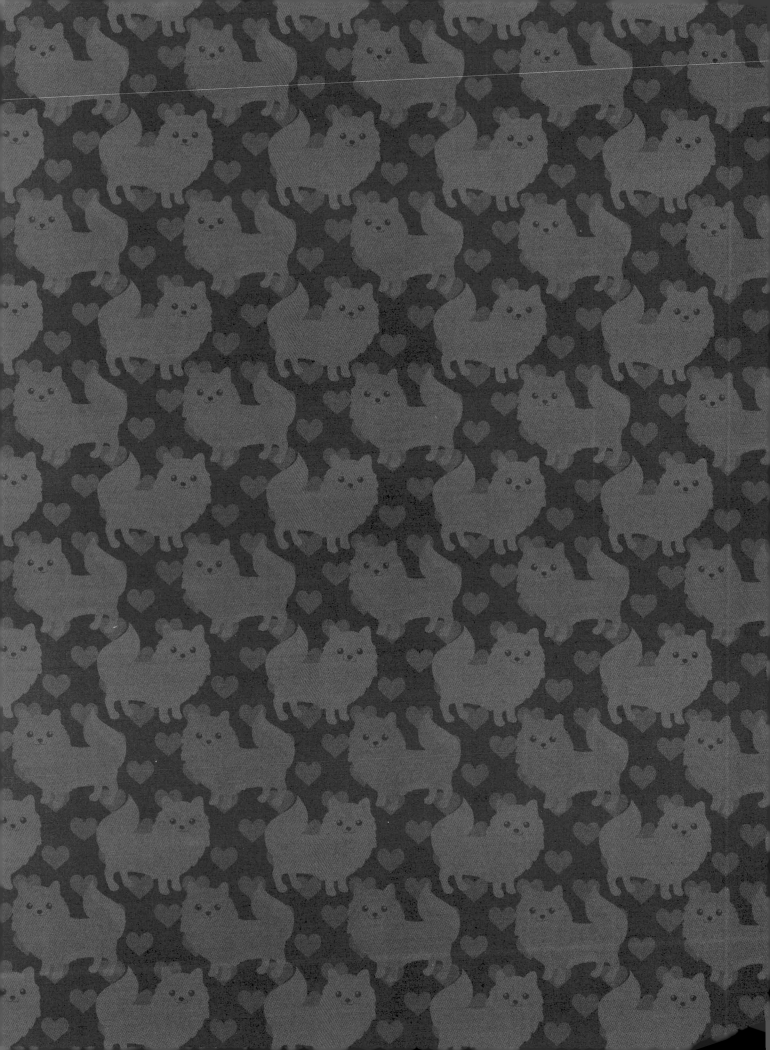

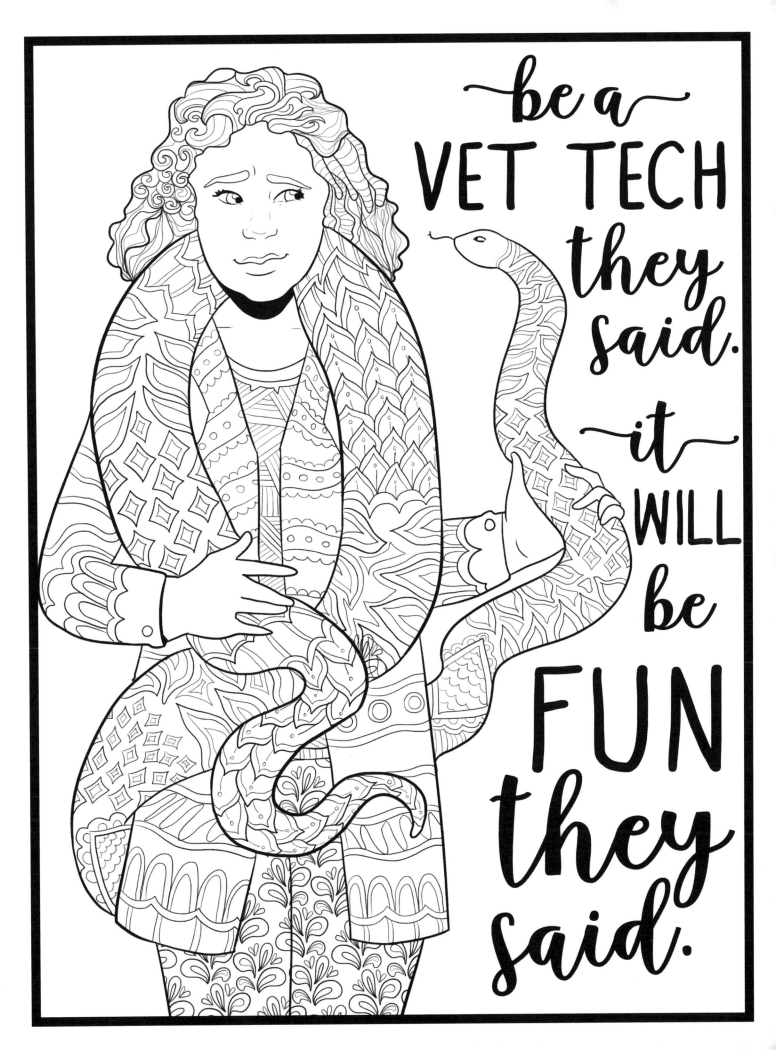

BE SURE TO FOLLOW US ON SOCIAL MEDIA FOR THE LATEST NEWS, SNEAK PEEKS, & GIVEAWAYS

@PapeterieBleu

Papeterie Bleu

@PapeterieBleu

ADD YOURSELF TO OUR MONTHLY NEWSLETTER FOR FREE DIGITAL DOWNLOADS AND DISCOUNT CODES

www.papeteriebleu.com/newsletter

CHECK OUT OUR OTHER BOOKS!

www.papeteriebleu.com

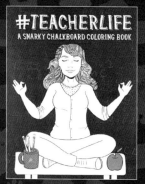 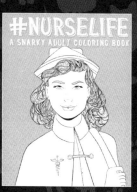 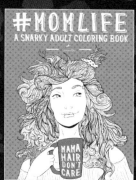 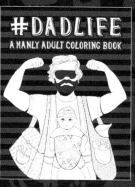 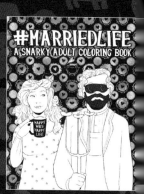

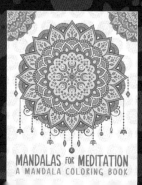 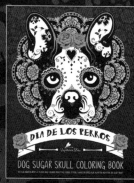 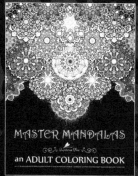 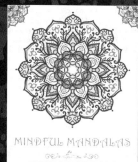 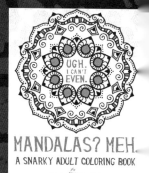

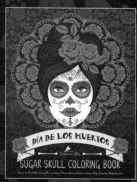 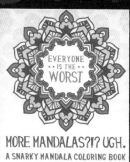 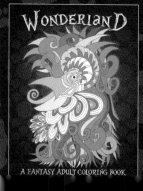 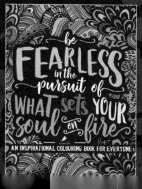 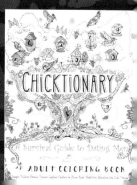

CHECK OUT OUR OTHER BOOKS!

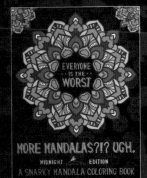
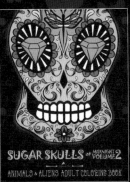
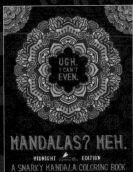

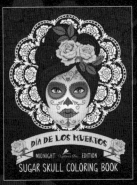
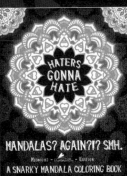
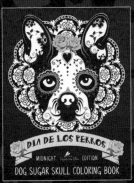
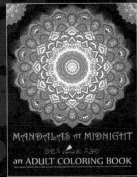
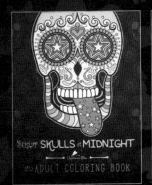
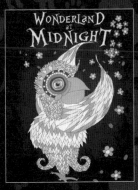
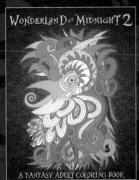
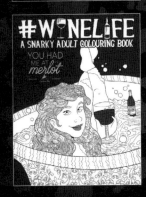
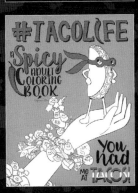
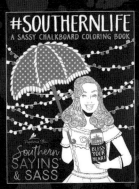
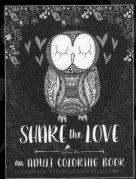
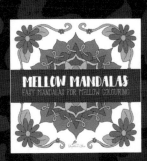

CHECK OUT OUR OTHER BOOKS!

www.papeteriebleu.com

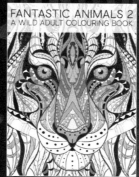

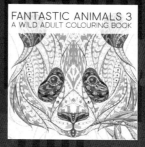

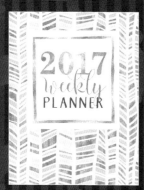

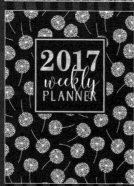

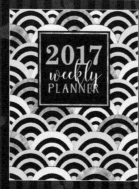

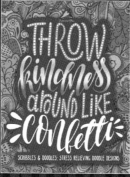

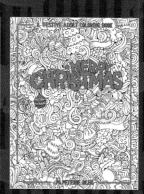

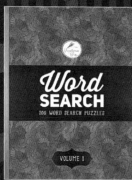

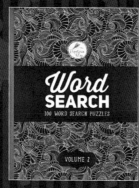

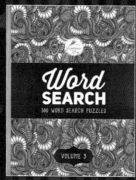

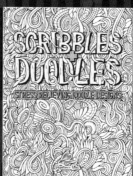

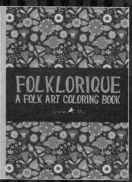

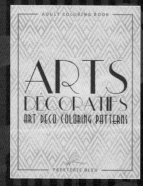

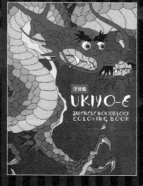

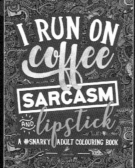

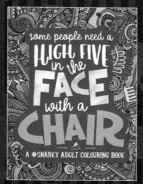

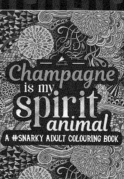

CPSIA information can be obtained at www.ICGtesting.com
Printed in the USA
BVIW120908040920
587919BV00010B/129